Managed Health Care Simplified:

A Glossary *of* Terms

Michael S. Austrin, M.A.

Strategic Planning, BJC Health System, St. Louis, Missouri.
Formerly consultant in healthcare and managed care.
Formerly Strategic Planning, RightCHOICE Managed Care, Inc.
(dba Alliance Blue Cross Blue Shield)
St. Louis, Missouri.

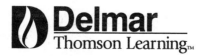

Africa • Australia • Canada • Denmark • Japan • Mexico • New Zealand • Philippines
Puerto Rico • Singapore • Spain • United Kingdom • United States

Delmar Staff:

Business Unit Director: William Brottmiller
Acquisitions Editor: Marion Walmar
Development Editor: Jill Rembetski
Editorial Assistant: Penny Cartwright
Executive Marketing Manager: Dawn Gerain
Channel Manager: Jaymee McRee
Art/Design Coordinator: Rich Killar
Cover Design: Charles Cummings
 Advertising/Art Inc.

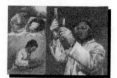

Delmar

ALLIED HEALTH
.Com

Library of Congress Cataloging-in-Publication Data

Austrin, Michael S.
  Managed health care simplified : a glossary of terms / Michael S. Austrin.
    p. cm.
  ISBN 0-7668-2078-5
  1. Managed care plans (Medical care)--Dictionaries. 2. Managed care plans (Medical care)--Acronyms. I. Title.
RA413 .A86 1999
362.1'04258'03--dc21

This book is dedicated to my wife Linda,
and our children Brian, Bradley and Brandon.

PREFACE

Managed care has a language all its own that, at times, can be puzzling. This book developed from my own frustration in trying to deal with a dizzying array of terms, acronyms and abbreviations. Managed care is an unusual environment with terms continuously being invented and defined. It is this type of setting where such terms as "incentive" have been modified into "incentivize."

Since managed care is a component of health care and, as such, not its own industry, its language needs to be documented to avoid confusion over the meaning of terms. Its terminology is unique since it is partially the language of health care combined with its own "special" business language. Consequently, it has created confusion not only for the layman, but also for those employed in health care. Further, managed care has wide variations in the definitions and usage of these terms. What I have attempted to do is bring together a base language. Variations will occur depending on the region, health plan, hospital, provider, medical school, nursing program, etc.

This book is straightforward with all terms listed in alphabetical order, and abbreviations and acronyms cross-referenced to their definitions. There are about 2,000 terms in the glossary; all are used in health insurance, health systems, hospitals, managed care organizations, physician offices, etc. Since managed care is so tightly linked to health care, it was necessary to include many health care terms to aid the reader's understanding of various managed care concepts. Excluded are those terms not related to managed care or those that would not further the reader's understanding. Cross-references are used extensively to help in comprehension, as well as for comparisons between terms. The appendices contain listings of journals, newsletters and magazines that cover the managed care industry, as well as listings of major associations and useful Internet sites.

My hope is that this book will serve as a tool for learning as well as for reference.

Michael S. Austrin

ACKNOWLEDGMENTS

I would like to thank the following people for their ideas, encouragement and input. Without their assistance, this book would have been much more difficult to complete.

I gratefully acknowledge Miriam G. Austrin, B.A., R.N. and Harvey R. Austrin, Ph.D., authors of *Learning Medical Terminology* (Mosby); Diane A. Klein, M.S., B.M.E., M.P.H., a specialist in Public Health and Wellness; F. James Grogan, Pharm. D., Executive Director of Pharmacy Benefit Designs and a specialist in pharmacy insurance programs; Walter Guller, a professional in managed care administration and insurance issues; Dora Lee Clark, an expert in quality improvement; Karen Roth, R.N. an expert in health care industry analysis; and Jerry Conlon, an employee benefits specialist and an expert on managed care.

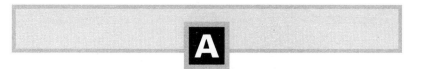

A

AAAASF – *See American Association for Accreditation of Ambulatory Surgery Facilities, Inc.*

AAAHC – *See Accreditation Association for Ambulatory Healthcare.*

AAHP – *See American Association of Health Plans.*

AAPCC – *See adjusted average per capita cost.*

AAPPO – *See American Association of Preferred Provider Organizations.*

ABMT – *See autologous bone marrow transplant.*

abstract – *See discharge summary.*

abuse – Improper or excessive use of program benefits or services by providers or consumers. Abuse can occur when services are used which are excessive or unnecessary; which are not the appropriate treatment for the patient's condition; when less expensive treatment would be as effective; or when billing or charging does not conform to requirements.

Abuse is differentiated from fraud, which is defined as deliberate deceit used by providers or consumers to 1) obtain payment for services not delivered or received, or 2) claim program eligibility.

ACAAI – *See American College of Allergy, Asthma and Immunology.*

Academy of Managed Care Pharmacy (AMCP) – An organization that represents pharmacists who work for managed care pharmacy organizations.

accelerated payment – Temporary partial advance of funds to providers due to temporary delays in payments on claims.

access – The ability to obtain medical care where and with whom one wants it. The term "access" is used when health plans talk about their networks. Access is determined by such components as the availability of medical services and their acceptability to the patient; the location of health care facilities; transportation; hours of operation; and cost of care. Since it involves many components, access is difficult to measure operationally. Still, many health plans attempt to find the perfect balance between size of network (how many doctors and hospitals), cost of health coverage (premium rates), and location of health care facilities (geographic vs. demographic).

A

access fee – The per member per month (PMPM) fee paid by a health insurer to a network to use that network of providers (physicians, hospitals, etc.). In layman's terms, access fee may be thought of as a rental fee; that is, the insurer is renting the use of a provider network for its members. *See per member per month.*

accidental bodily injury – Injury to the body as a result of an accident.

Accidental Death and Dismemberment Coverage (ADD) – A plan that provides benefits in the event of loss of life, limb, or eyesight as the result of an accident. ADD is usually a supplementary benefit to regular group term life insurance coverage.

accommodation – Type of hospital room (e.g., private, semiprivate, ICU, etc.).

accountable health plan (AHP) – A health care delivery organization that integrates the financial, clinical, managerial and preventive aspects of health care delivery. By linking hospitals, physicians and payers through contractual and financial arrangements, AHPs assume responsibility and risk for delivering medical care to a specific community. Since it includes both payers and providers, the AHP produces a network which provides coordinated and comprehensive care with continuous monitoring of quality, cost, health outcomes and patient satisfaction. The plans generally have some incentive to develop preventive programs and emphasize wellness; and physicians and other providers either own, work for, or contract with these health plans.

When an AHP operates one or more health insurance benefit products, or a managed care organization acquires a large scale medical delivery component, it qualifies as an accountable health system or accountable health plan.

Accountable health plans are also known as integrated delivery system (IDS), integrated health system (IHS), integrated health delivery system (IHDS), community accountable healthcare network (CAHN), integrated service networks (ISN), health purchasing alliance (HPA), community care network (CCN) and organized delivery systems.

accreditation – A "stamp of approval" given by an agency or organization to a health care plan that meets their predetermined standards. Accreditation is usually given by a private organization created for the purpose of assuring the public of the quality of the accredited, such as the Joint Commission on Accreditation of Healthcare Organizations. Accreditation standards and individual performance

A

with respect to such standards are not always available to the public. In some situations, public governments recognize accreditation as the basis of licensure. Public or private payment programs often require accreditation as a condition of payment for covered services. For HMOs, the leading accreditation agency is the National Committee for Quality Assurance (NCQA).

Accreditation standards and individual performance with respect to such standards (e.g., JCAHO) are available to the public if they wish to access this information.

Accreditation Association for Ambulatory Health Care (AAAHC) – An organization that offers accreditation for ambulatory care organizations.

accredited hospital – A hospital whose quality of care meets standards set by the Joint Commission on Accreditation of Healthcare Organizations. *See Joint Commission on Accreditation of Healthcare Organizations.*

accrete – A Medicare term meaning the addition of new recipients to a health plan.

accrual – The amount of money that is set aside to cover health care expenses or costs. The accrual is a health plan's estimate of what medical expenses will be incurred and is actuarially based on a combination of data from the authorization system, demographic assumptions, the claims system and the plan's prior history.

accrue – To recognize and report an event or transaction in the time period to which its effect relates.

accumulation – The total number of utilized services within a dollar-limited or visit-limited covered benefit.

accumulation period – A specified period of time (e.g., 90 days) during which the insured person must incur eligible medical expenses at least equal to the deductible amount in order to establish a benefit period. Accumulation period applies to a major medical or comprehensive medical plan.

ACER – Annual Contractor Evaluation Report. A Medicare term.

ACF – *See alternative care facility.*

acquisition cost – The health insurance or managed care company's immediate cost of selling, underwriting and issuing a new health insurance policy. This includes administrative costs, brokers' commissions, advertising and medical fees.

A

ACR – *See adjusted community rating.*

active – Status currently in effect. May refer to a group or individual subscriber.

actively-at-work – Describes a health plan's requirement that health care coverage not go into effect until the employee's first day of work on or after the effective date of coverage. Actively-at-work may also apply to dependents disabled on the effective date.

Activities of Daily Living (ADLs) – An individual's daily habits such as bathing, dressing and eating. ADLs are often used as an assessment tool to determine one's ability to function at home or in a less restricted environment of care.

actual acquisition cost – A prescription drug program term meaning the actual cost of a drug to the pharmacy or to the managed care organization that is associated with the pharmacist.

actual charge – The amount a physician or other health care practitioner actually bills a patient for a particular medical service or procedure. The actual charge may differ from the customary, prevailing and reasonable charges. *See customary, prevailing and reasonable.*

actuarial – The statistical calculations used to determine a managed care company's rates and premiums based on projections of utilization and cost for a defined customer population.

actuarial assumptions – The assumptions (educated guesses) that an actuary uses in calculating the expected costs and revenues of the health plan. Examples include utilization rates, age and sex mix of enrollees, and cost for medical services.

actuarial soundness – The requirement that the development of capitation rates (fixed rates) meet commonly accepted actuarial (statistical calculations) principles and rules. *See capitation, actuary and actuarial.*

actuary – A professional trained in the science of mathematical probabilities who specializes in the evaluation of short-term and long-term risks. For insurance purposes, an actuary is a person who determines insurance policy rates, reserves and dividends. Actuaries are vital in the development of physician capitation rates. *See capitation.*

acuity – A measure of patient sickness severity, used to establish nurse staffing needs.

A

acute care – Short-term health care and treatment provided to patients who require concentrated and continuous observation. The patient is treated for an acute (immediate and severe) episode of illness, for the treatment of injuries related to accidents or other trauma, or during recovery from surgery. Acute care is usually given in a hospital by specialized personnel for 30 days or less. Compare to chronic care. *See also acute disease.*

acute care services – Coordinated services related to the examination, diagnosis, care and treatment of immediate and severe episodes of illness.

acute disease – A disease which is characterized by a single episode of fairly short duration from which the patient returns to his normal or previous state and level of activity. Acute diseases are distinguished from chronic diseases, where by the patient has reached his or her optimal level of functioning. For example, a patient with chronic obstructive pulmonary disease (COPD) that lives with the disease with proper care and treatment.

ADA – *See American Dental Association.* ADA may also stand for Americans with Disabilities Act or American Diabetic Association.

additional diagnosis – Any diagnosis, other than the principal diagnosis, that describes a condition for which a patient is receiving treatment, or for which the attending physician considers further study justifiable.

additions (ADDS) – New subscriber contracts or members.

ADEA – *See Age Discrimination in Employment Act of 1967.*

adequate rates – Rates that generate premiums sufficient to cover incurred claims, operating costs, risk charges and contingency reserve requirements.

adjudication – The process a payer uses to decide whether to pay or reject an insurance claim and how much to pay based on benefit plan provisions. This includes membership validation, liability determination and previous utilization history of the participant.

adjusted average per capita cost (AAPCC) – The Health Care Financing Administration's (HCFA) best estimate of the amount of money needed for care of Medicare recipients in a given area under fee-for-service. The AAPCC is made up of 122 different rate cells (classifications); 120 of them are factored for age, sex, Medicaid eligibility, institutional status and whether a person has both Part A (hospital) and Part B (physicians) of Medicare. HCFA uses the

A

AAPCCs to make monthly payments to risk and cost contractors.

adjusted community rating (ACR) – A method for setting health insurance rates based on a group's specific demographics and prior health experience. Also known as factored rating and community rating by class (CRC). *See community rating and prospective rating.* Compare to modified community rating (MCR).

adjusted drug benefit list – A small number of medications often prescribed to long-term patients. The list can be modified from time to time by a health plan, HCFA or a 3rd party administrator. Also called a drug maintenance list. *See also drug formulary or formulary.*

adjusted payment rate (APR) – The amount of money that the Health Care Financing Administration (HCFA) will pay Medicare risk HMOs to cover a Medicare beneficiary. The rate is derived from the adjusted average per capita cost (AAPCC) based on health risk factors for the beneficiaries. *See adjusted average per capita cost* (AAPCC).

adjustment – A change made to a paid claim due to a processor error, policy change, physician billing error or plan problem.

adjustment reasons – A list of coded explanations used as a reference guide to explain changes made to a paid claim. The codes provide an explanation about almost any service reported and eliminate the need for a separate letter of explanation.

administration – Most often refers to claims processing and adjudication, but may also be used to describe all of the administrative costs in the management of a health plan, such as member eligibility verification, benefit interpretation, provider relations, utilization management, capitation accounting, actuarial analysis, case management, coordination of benefits and peer review.

administrative costs – *See administrative expenses.*

administrative expenses – A health plan's costs associated with doing business, including such costs as marketing, medical underwriting, commissions, premium collection, claims processing, quality assurance, risk management and utilization review. Also called administrative costs or administrative loading.

administrative guidelines – The interpretation of the health plan document as approved by the plan administrator. The health plan document is a written description of a health plan's benefits and explanations of filing claims, payment of claims, deductibles, prescription drug plan, coordination of benefits, administrative rules, etc. The plan administrator is responsible for the actual adminis-

A

tration of the health plan.

administrative loading – *See administrative expenses.*

Administrative Services Organization (ASO) – An organization that performs administrative services such as billing, practice management and marketing for a self-funded entity, but not risk-bearing services, such as claims processing and stop-loss coverage (protection from unexpected financial loss). *See also third party administrator* (TPA) *and stop-loss.*

administrative services only (ASO) – Self-funding arrangement in which a third party (e.g., insurance company or other entity) performs administrative services only (e.g., billing, practice management, marketing, etc.) for a self-funded group (usually an employer). The group assumes any and all risk for the cost of health care services provided to its members. ASO may include or exclude some services depending on the contract.

administrator – The entity responsible for processing health care claims. *See third party administrator.*

admission – The process of registering a patient for inpatient or outpatient hospital services. For inpatients, a patient is provided with room, board and continuous nursing service in a hospital or facility where patients generally stay at least overnight. For outpatient admissions, a patient is provided with room, board and continuous nursing service in a hospital or facility where patients generally do not stay overnight. Particularly in hospitals, it is usually expected that outpatient admissions will be sent home the same day. Outpatient services are usually considered the same as ambulatory services.

The day of admission is the actual day that the hospital or medical center assigned a register number to the patient. Admission data include direct admissions, direct admissions from the emergency room and transfer-in patients from other medical treatment facilities. Newborns are reported separately and excluded from the admission data.

admission and disposition report – A daily hospital report reflecting patients gained and lost (census), and changes in status and numerical strengths of transient patients and boarders.

admission certification – A form of medical care review that assures only those patients who need hospital care are admitted, without unnecessary delay and with proper planning of the hospital stay.

A

Certification can be done before admission (preadmission) or shortly after (concurrent). Length-of-stay for the patient's diagnosed problem is usually assigned and certified.

Admissions/1000 – *See admissions per* 1000.

Admissions Per 1000 (APT) – The method of comparing the number of hospital admissions for defined populations. Basically, it is the number of hospital admissions for a population divided by the number of persons in that population, with the result multiplied by 1000.

Specifically, admissions per 1000 is calculated by taking the total number of inpatient and/or outpatient admissions from a specific group (e.g., employer group, HMO population at risk, etc.) for a specific period of time, usually one year. This figure is divided by the average number of covered members in that group during the same period, with the result multiplied by 1000.

APT can be calculated for behavioral health or any disease in the aggregate and by modality of treatment (e.g., inpatient, residential, partial hospitalization, etc.). Such measures are commonly used by managed care entities to evaluate utilization management performance.

admission wire – A Blue Cross and Blue Shield term meaning a formal notification sent by a host plan to the home plan that one of their members has been admitted into a plan hospital in the host plan's area and requesting membership information. *See approval wire.*

admitting diagnosis – The condition identified to be responsible for the patient's admission to a hospital.

admitting physician – The physician responsible for arranging a patient's admission to a hospital or other inpatient health facility. The physician may maintain control over the patient's care or may transfer the patient to a specialist, depending on the nature of the illness.

ADS – *See alternate delivery system.*

adult day care – Refers to care for seniors by a professional staff available during the day, either in the home or at a facility. Services may include therapy, rehabilitation and nursing care.

adult foster care (AFC) – Refers to assistance provided to individuals over the age of 18 who are no longer able to live alone and care for themselves, but do not need daily nursing supervision. Adult fos-

A

ter care is provided on a 24-hour basis in a facility with a home-like environment. AFC homes are small, generally with 5 to 10 residents, and are differentiated from other residential care settings by both the size of the homes and the family nature of the care setting.

AFC homes fall under the category of assisted living centers, providing general supervision and personal care services for individuals who require minimal assistance in the Activities of Daily Living (ADLs), require supervision or monitoring with the self-administration of medications, or require supervision or monitoring of self-treatment of a physical disorder. ADLs include sleeping, dressing, bathing, eating, brushing teeth, combing hair, etc. AFC homes are usually licensed and regulated by the state they reside in. Also called domiciliary care. *See assisted living center* (ALC) *and Activities of Daily Living* (ADL).

advance check – Payment sent to a provider that precedes filing of a claim.

advance directive – Refers to a patient's wishes regarding continuation or withdrawal of treatment if the situation arises whereby he/she lacks decision-making capacity. Advance directives are arranged prior to admission to a hospital. Examples include do-not-resuscitate orders (DNR) and a living will, which make it clear that the patient does not wish life-sustaining measures to be used in the event of either poor quality of life or a hopeless illness.

adverse selection – Describes the situation in which a plan has a disproportionate percentage of members who are prone to higher than average utilization of benefits because of existing higher health risk conditions. This may be because the plan attracted members who are sicker than the general population or because the member base is sicker than was anticipated when the budget for medical costs was developed. Whatever the reason, adverse selection is not good for payers since the higher utilization usually drives health costs above those covered by the capitation rate. As such, adverse selection is also used to describe occasions when premiums do not cover costs due to the above situation.

AFC – *See adult foster care.*

AFDC – *See Aid to Families with Dependent Children.*

affiliated health care provider – *See participating provider.*

affiliated hospital – A hospital that has an established relationship with another health entity, usually a medical school.

A

age break – The grouping of age categories for rating purposes. For example, females age 18 to 25.

Age Discrimination in Employment Act of 1967 (ADEA) – As amended in 1978, ADEA requires employers with 200 or more employees to offer older active employees under age 70 and who are eligible for Medicare (and their spouses if they are also under age 70), the same health insurance coverage that is provided to younger employees.

age limits – Stipulated minimum and maximum ages below and above which the health insurance or managed care company will not accept applications or may not renew policies.

age/sex factor – A measurement used in actuarial underwriting which uses the age and sex risk of medical costs of one population relative to another population. *See actuarial.*

age/sex rates (ASR) – A method of structuring payments or premiums based on each member's age and sex. Age/sex rates are a set of rates for a given group product broken out by age and sex categories, used to calculate premiums for group billing purposes. ASR is often preferred over single and family rating in small groups because it automatically adjusts to demographic changes within the group. Also called table rates.

age/sex rating – *See age/sex rates.*

aged – For Social Security purposes, a term used for people 65 years and older whose income and resources are within supplemental security income (SSI) limitations.

Agency for Health Care Policy and Research (AHCPR) – U.S. Public Health Service responsible for enhancing the quality, appropriateness and effectiveness of health care services.

agent – *See broker.*

aggregate indemnity – The maximum dollar amount payable for any disability, period of disability, or covered service under an insurance policy.

aggregate stop loss – A mechanism used by an insurer to relieve the amount of liability for claims in excess of the amount expected for the contract year. *See stop loss.*

AGPA – *See American Medical Group Association.*

AHA – *See American Hospital Association.*

A

AHCA – *See American Health Care Association.*

AHCPR – Agency for Health Care Policy and Research.

Aid to Families with Dependent Children (AFDC) – According to the U.S. Census Bureau, AFDC is "a program administered and funded by Federal and State governments to provide financial assistance to needy families. In an average State, more than half (55 percent) of the total cost of AFDC payments are funded by the Federal government. The States provide the balance of these payments, manage the program, and determine who receives benefits and how much they get." Children who qualify for AFDC assistance also receive Medicaid benefits.

To be eligible to receive AFDC payments, a family must have a dependent child who is:

- Under age 18 and living with them.
- Deprived of financial support from one of his or her parents due to the parent's death, continued absence, or incapacity (including unemployment).
- A resident of the state they live in and a U.S. citizen or an alien who is permanently and lawfully residing in the U.S.

alignment of incentives – Describes financial arrangements between physicians and hospitals that allow both parties to share in the risks and rewards of controlling costs and increasing revenue. *See incentives.*

all clause deductible – Application of a deductible under a health care plan to all covered expenses incurred by a person as a result of the same or related causes within a given time (accumulation period).

all inclusive rate – Payment rates to providers that include ancillary services (e.g., laboratory tests or x-rays) plus routine services (e.g., full physical or check-up).

allocation – Distributing organizational costs (financial, operational and personnel) according to responsibilities assumed, usage or other rational measures. Allocation is primarily used to pass overhead costs to different departments.

allopathy – A system of medicine based on the theory that successful therapy depends on creating a condition antagonistic to or incompatible with the condition to be treated. For example, antibiotic drugs are given to patients to fight diseases caused by the organisms to which the drugs are antagonistic. Allopathy is the predominant system in the United States, and its practitioners are

A

Doctors of Medicine (MDs). Compare to homeopathy and osteopathy.

allowable charge – Charges for services rendered or supplies furnished by a health care provider that qualify as covered expenses under a health plan. Allowable charges are reimbursable under a payment formula from the health plan. In general, uncovered expenses would include any expenditure that the health plan deems unnecessary in the efficient delivery of health care; for instance, uncovered services or luxury accommodations.

allowable costs – *See maximum allowable and allowable charge.*

allowed amount – *See maximum allowable.*

allowed charges – *See allowable charge.*

All Patient-Diagnosis Related Groups (APDRG or AP-DRG) – An enhancement of the original DRGs, developed by 3M Health Information Systems and designed to apply to a population broader than that of Medicare beneficiaries, who are predominately older individuals. The APDRG set includes groupings for pediatric and maternity cases as well as of services for HIV-related conditions and other special cases.

all-payer system – A system in which prices for health services and payment methods are the same, regardless of who is paying. In an all-payer system, federal or state government, a private insurer, a self-insured employer plan, an individual or any other payer could pay the same rates. The uniform fee bars health care providers from shifting costs from one payer to another. *See cost shifting.*

alternate financing mechanism – *See alternative funding mechanism.*

alternative care facility (ACF) – An assisted living facility for seniors who do not require nursing care. Most ACFs offer private and semi-private rooms to residents and are conveniently located to shopping and entertainment facilities.

alternative delivery system (ADS) – All forms of health care delivery other than traditional fee-for-service (FFS). Alternative delivery systems include prepaid group practice, individual practice associations (IPA), preferred provider organizations (PPO), point of service (POS), and Health Maintenance Organizations (HMO).

ADS can also mean health care services provided outside of an inpatient, acute-care hospital. For instance, skilled and intermediary nursing facilities, hospice programs, behavioral health centers and home health care.

A

alternative funding mechanism – Generally a financing mechanism designed to provide the account with a more favorable cash flow. Some examples include self-funding and deferred premiums.

alternative medicine – Alternative medicine includes such nontraditional therapies as acupuncture, massage, mind/body therapies, chiropractic, nutritional and herbal medicine, diet, exercise, stress management and meditation. Many health insurance companies and managed care organizations now provide coverage for a few of these alternative therapies. The National Institute of Health's Office of Alternative Medicine has identified and categorized over 300 different alternative approaches into the following fields:

- Alternative Systems of Medical Practice—Health care ranging from self-care according to folk principles, to care rendered in an organized healthcare system based on alternative traditions or practices.
- Bioelectromagnetic Applications—The study of how living organisms interact with electromagnetic (EM) fields.
- Diet, Nutrition, Lifestyle Changes—The knowledge of how to prevent illness, maintain health, and reverse the effects of chronic disease through dietary or nutritional intervention.
- Herbal Medicine—Employing plant and plant products from folk medicine traditions for pharmacological use.
- Manual Healing—Using touch and manipulation with the hands as a diagnostic and therapeutic tool.
- Mind-Body Control—Exploring the mind's capacity to affect the body, based on traditional medical systems that make use of the interconnectedness of mind and body.
- Pharmacological & Biological Treatments—Drugs and vaccines not yet accepted by mainstream medicine.

AMA – *See American Medical Association.*

ambulatory care – Medical, surgical, or diagnostic services provided on an outpatient basis. That is, health care services provided without the patient being admitted or requiring an overnight stay. Includes the services of hospital outpatient departments, physicians' offices, dentist's offices, home health care and ambulatory care centers. Also known as outpatient care.

ambulatory care clinic – An entity or unit of a medical or dental treatment facility that is organized and staffed to provide medical treatment in a particular specialty and/or subspecialty, and holds regular hours in a designated place. *See ambulatory care facility.*

ambulatory care group (ACG) – *See ambulatory patient group.*

A

ambulatory care evaluation – Peer review to assure the quality of medical care, services and procedures provided to ambulatory patients. A function of the local medical society or other organization authorized by the medical society, in a geographically defined locality which incorporates the concepts of utilization review and medical audit.

ambulatory care facility – A freestanding or hospital-based facility providing preventative diagnosis, emergency therapeutic services, elective surgery or other treatment not requiring an overnight stay. *See ambulatory surgical center.*

ambulatory patient – A patient with the ability to walk or ambulate in a wheelchair.

ambulatory patient care groups – *See ambulatory patient classifications.*

ambulatory patient classification groups – *See ambulatory patient classifications.*

ambulatory patient classifications (APC) – The Balanced Budget Act of 1997 (BBA) authorizes the Health Care Financing Administration (HCFA) to implement a Medicare prospective payment system (PPS) for hospital outpatient services, certain Part B services furnished to inpatients who have no Part A coverage, and partial hospitalization services furnished by community mental health centers. Excluded are items and services covered by another Medicare fee schedule, such as laboratory and therapy, and certain services that are appropriate and safe only in an inpatient setting (e.g., CABG).

A major component of the PPS is the ambulatory payment classifications (APCs) currently consisting of: 348 groups of 8,000+ outpatient services made up of the following:

- 46 groups of significant procedures, such as radiation oncology
- 136 groups of surgical procedures
- 121 groups of medical visits
- 45 groups of ancillary services, such as x-rays

HCFA is also considering additional separate APCs for high-cost drugs, technology and supportive cancer therapies. The services within each group are related clinically and in terms of their resource use. Hospitals receive the same PPS rate for procedures in the same APC. HCFA could change procedure APC assignments if there is evidence that a reassignment would improve either the clinical or resource consumption of the group(s). Any changes in the APC groups must be budget neutral.

A

Ambulatory patient classifications are also called ambulatory payment classes, ambulatory patient classification groups and ambulatory patient care groups.

ambulatory patient group (APG) – Similar to DRGs (diagnosis-related group), APGs are used to categorize ambulatory patients into case types to provide a pricing mechanism for outpatient services. Also called ambulatory care group and ambulatory visit group. In 2000, APGs were replaced with ambulatory patient classifications (APC), authorized by the 1997 passing of the Balanced Budget Act (BBA). *See ambulatory patient classifications.*

ambulatory payment classes – *See ambulatory patient classifications.*

ambulatory surgery – Surgery performed on an outpatient basis, where the patient goes home the same day the procedure is performed.

ambulatory surgery center (ASC) – An operating facility, either freestanding or hospital-based, where outpatient surgery is performed. The ASC is primarily for an intermediate level of surgical care for procedures that are too complex to be done in a physician's office but do not require inpatient hospitalization. Also called surgi-center and ambulatory surgical center.

The ASC is a public or private establishment that:

- has an organized medical staff of physicians,
- has permanent facilities that are equipped and operated primarily for the purpose of performing surgical procedures,
- has continuous physician service and registered professional nursing services whenever a patient is in the facility,
- does not provide services or other accommodations for patients to stay overnight, and
- is licensed as an ambulatory surgery center by the state in which it operates.

ambulatory surgery program – A facility program for the performance of elective surgical procedures on patients who are admitted and discharged on the day the procedure is performed.

ambulatory utilization review (AUR) – Utilization review performed for ambulatory patients. *See utilization review.*

ambulatory visit – A visit to a physician, clinic or specialty service by a patient who is not admitted to a hospital.

ambulatory visit group (AVG) – *See ambulatory patient group.*

AMCP – *See Academy of Managed Care Pharmacy.*

A

AMCPA – American Managed Care Pharmacy Association.

AMCRA – American Managed Care and Review Association. *See* AAHP.

amendment – A legal document attached to a contract whereby the scope of its terms are either increased or restricted.

American Association for Accreditation of Ambulatory Surgery Facilities, Inc. (AAAASF) – An organization that offers accreditation for outpatient care organizations.

American Association of Health Plans (AAHP) – An association formed by the uniting of the Group Health Association of America (GHAA) and the American Managed Care and Review Association (AMCRA).

American Association of Preferred Provider Organizations (AAPPO) – A not-for-profit association of network-based managed health care entities and affiliate organizations that assists its members' efforts to improve the quality, accessibility and affordability of health services.

American College of Allergy, Asthma and Immunology (ACAAI) – An organization of allergists-immunologists and related health care professionals dedicated to quality patient care through research, advocacy and professional and public education.

American Dental Association (ADA) – A nonprofit organization dedicated to the advancement of dentistry and the dental profession.

American Group Practice Association (AGPA) – *See American Medical Group Association* (AMGA).

American Health Care Association (AHCA) – A federation of 50 state health organizations, together representing nearly 12,000 non-profit and for-profit assisted living, nursing facility, long-term care, and subacute care providers that care for more than one million elderly and disabled individuals nationally.

American Hospital Association (AHA) – A voluntary association of hospitals organized for the purpose of helping hospitals provide better patient care.

American Managed Care and Review Association (AMCRA) – *See American Association of Health Plans* (AAHP).

American Managed Care Pharmacy Association (AMCPA) – An organization representing managed care pharmacy organizations, including mail-order pharmacies.

A

American Medical Association (AMA) – A public service organization composed of state and territorial medical societies dedicated to the advancement of science and medicine and the betterment of the public health welfare.

American Medical Group Association (AMGA) – Formed from the merger of the American Group Practice Association (AGPA) and the Unified Medical Group Association (UMGA). The AMGA is an association of physicians in group practices that provides its members with continuing medical education, legislative representation and outcomes measurement programs.

amount billed – The value of the health care service provided to a patient as defined on the claim submitted by the provider.

amount, duration and scope – How a Medicaid benefit is defined and limited in a state's Medicaid plan. Since each state defines these parameters, Medicaid plans vary from state to state in what is actually covered.

AMPS – *See Automated Medicaid Payment System.*

anchor group – Large multi-disciplinary, multi-specialty behavioral group practices tapped by health insurance or managed care companies to handle intake, referral and treatment of patients. These groups draw the bulk of referrals under managed care contracts and carry most of the clinical risk. Also called key groups or core groups. *See carve-out.*

ancillary services – Services that assist and augment the talents of attending physicians and dentists in diagnosing and treating patients. These services are available to a patient apart from physician and general nursing care, and generally do not have primary responsibility for the clinical management of patients. Examples include physical or respiratory therapy, laboratory tests and x-rays.

anesthesia – Partial or complete loss of sensation with or without loss of consciousness as a result of illness, disease, or use of an administered anesthetic agent.

anesthesia minutes of service – The elapsed time during any procedure involving an anesthesiologist and/or anesthetist multiplied by the number of anesthesiologists and/or anesthetists, including residents and student nurse anesthetists (when replacing a person trained in anesthesia), participating in the procedure.

anesthesiologist – A physician who specializes in the administration of anesthetics for the purpose of eliminating the sensation of pain, usually during surgical procedures.

anesthesiology – Science involving the administration of anesthesia, drugs or gas to produce the loss of sensation in a patient, and nerve blocks.

anesthetist – A person who specializes in the administration of anesthetics during surgical procedures. *See certified registered nurse anesthetist* (CRNA).

anniversary – *See anniversary date.*

anniversary date –
1. The yearly observance of the date an individual or group benefit program became effective. For example, if March 1st is the first day of effective coverage of an employer's health plan, then March 1st is considered the anniversary date.
2. Date on which an employee enters a new year of employment.

annual completion factor – Factor to adjust 12 months of incurred and paid claims to 12 months of expected incurred claims. *See incurred claims and expected incurred claims.*

annual deductible – *See deductible.*

annual maximum – The maximum dollar amount an insurance company will cover on all claims incurred in one year for an insured party, as defined in a benefit plan.

annuity – A contract that provides an income for a stated time period or for an annuitant's lifetime.

any willing provider (AWP) – State laws that require managed care plans to accept any and all health care providers that meet their terms and conditions. This includes agreeing to the managed care organization's reimbursement rates and utilization guidelines. Specific AWP definitions vary from state to state, but most include due process laws that impose requirements on how health care providers are selected and terminated from health plans.

APC – *See ambulatory patient classifications.*

APDRG or AP-DRG – *See all patient-diagnosis related groups.*

appeal review – A process that allows the enrollee or provider to request reconsideration of a benefit decision by a health plan. Appeals can be submitted to the health plan itself or the Department of Insurance of the state where the health plan is located. Appeals to self-insured plans are typically submitted to the

A

employer or U.S. Department of Labor.

application card – Form completed and signed by an applicant requesting coverage for which he/she is entitled.

appropriateness – Care for which the expected health benefit exceeds the expected negative consequences by a wide enough margin to justify treatment.

approval – Information given to a health care provider to indicate a health plan's acceptance of liability and the level of benefits applicable to the claim.

approval wire – A Blue Cross and Blue Shield term describing a formal notification that is sent to the host plan from the home plan after the home plan has received the admission wire and has verified membership information. Gives approval for specific number of days and contract benefits. *See admission wire.*

approved amount – *See maximum allowable.*

approved charge –
1. Charges approved for payment by private health plans.
2. Items that are likely to be reimbursed by an insurance or managed care company.
3. The limits of expenses that Medicare will pay in a given area of covered service.

approved health care facility, hospital or program – A facility, hospital or program authorized to provide health care services and allowed by a given health plan to provide services stipulated in contracts.

APR – *See adjusted payment rate.*

arrears – Billing subscribers for prior month's dues not paid.

ASC – *See ambulatory surgery center.*

ASO – *See administrative services only.*

asset – An economic resource that is expected to benefit the accounting entity and its activities in future accounting periods.

assigned risk – A risk which underwriters do not care to insure but which, because of state law or otherwise, must be insured; for instance, a person with hypertension seeking health insurance. Insuring assigned risks is usually handled through a group of insurers (such as all companies licensed to issue health insurance in the state) and individual assigned risks are assigned to the companies

A

in turn or in proportion of their share of the state's total health insurance business. Assignment of risks is less common in health insurance than it is in casualty insurance.

assignment – *See assignment of benefits.*

assignment of benefits – An agreement which a patient signs instructing the insurance company to pay the health care provider directly for services rendered. Assignment is used instead of direct payment by patient for the service for which he/she would receive reimbursement from public or private insurance programs.

Under Medicare, a provider who accepts assignment agrees not to bill Medicare beneficiaries for charges above the reasonable and customary charge allowed by Medicare. The provider accepts the Medicare program allowance as payment in full (except for coinsurance, copayment and deductible amounts required of the patient). As such, assignment of benefits protects the patient against liability for charges which the Medicare program will not recognize as reasonable.

assisted living – Care for people who need assistance with the Activities of Daily Living (ADL), want to live as independently as possible, and do not require constant care. (Activities of Daily Living include such things as eating, bathing, dressing, laundry, housekeeping and taking medications.) Assisted living exists to bridge the gap between independent living and nursing homes, and offers an intermediate level of long-term care ideal for seniors who are not ready for the expense and intensive level of care found in a nursing home.

assisted living center (ALC) – Facilities that care for people needing assistance with the Activities of Daily Living (ADL), who want to live as independently as possible, and do not require constant care. ALCs are similar to nursing homes but provide for more independence for their residents. They range in size from small homelike environments of about 3 to 15 residents (typically referred to as adult foster care or domiciliary care) to large, full-service communities with 600 to 800 residents. Services vary, but usually include meals, 24-hour emergency monitoring, supervision and dispensing of medications, socialization with peers and assistance with one or more ADLs.

Approximately 1 million Americans live in assisted-living centers. Assisted living is the generic term used, but it is also known as assisted living facility (ALF), adult foster care, domiciliary care, residential care, etc. *See assisted living, adult foster care* (AFC) *and Activities of Daily Living* (ADL).

assisted living facility (ALF) – *See assisted living center* (ALC).

association – A group of persons, usually trade or business groups, who have joined together for some special purpose or business.

attending physician – The physician in charge of the patient's care, who may or may not be the physician who admitted (admitting physician) the patient to the hospital. It is possible for a patient to have more than one attending physician providing treatment at the same time if the patient suffers from multiple medical conditions. Depending on the hospital, additional attending physicians may instead be called consulting physicians.

attrition rate – Disenrollment from a health plan expressed as a percentage of total membership. An HMO with 50,000 members which loses 1,000 members over a year experiences a 2% (two percent) annual attrition rate.

audiology – The study, examination and treatment of hearing defects, including the use of hearing aids and other therapy.

audit of provider treatment or charges – A qualitative or quantitative review of services rendered or proposed by a health provider. The review can be carried out in a number of ways: a comparison of patient records and claim form information, a patient questionnaire, a review of hospital and practitioner records, or a pre- or post-treatment clinical examination of a patient. Some audits may involve fee verification. The audit is sometimes thought of as the "first generation" managed care approach.

audit trail, visit – A retrospective validation of a patient's episode of care, resulting from a review of the records generated by the provider or clinic at the time the care was provided.

AUR – *See ambulatory utilization review.*

authenticate –
   1. To denote authorship of an entry made in a patient's medical or dental record by means of a written signature, identifiable initials or a personally used rubber stamp.
   2. The process of certifying copies as genuine.

authorization – The process of determining that a given service is medically appropriate and performed by the appropriate provider. Authorization is usually issued by the health plan or ultimate payer of claims. Also called prior authorization or pre-certification.

A

autologous bone marrow transplant (ABMT) – A cancer treatment for which the patient is his or her own bone marrow donor, as opposed to allogenic bone marrow transplant, where the donor is another person.

automated claims payment – A claim system involving the use of a computer in the adjudication of medical, dental or disability claims. The Automated Medicaid Payment System (AMPS) is an example.

Automated Medicaid Payment System (AMPS) – A claim system involving the use of a computer in the adjudication of Medicaid patient claims.

availability – When an individual can obtain appropriate health care at the time and place needed. More specifically, it is the supply of health care providers, services and resources in relation to the needs or demands of a given individual or community.

available hours – The hours for which pay is earned (regular, overtime and holiday), which are provided by the presence of an assigned employee for the performance of work or other medical mission needs.

available time – The hours worked or expended in support of health care.

average daily census – Average number of inpatients, excluding newborns, receiving care each day during a reported period.

average daily patient load—bassinet (ADPL-BASS) – The average number of live births in the hospital receiving care each day during a reported period. Bassinet ADPL is calculated by dividing the number of bassinet days during the period by the total number of days in the report period. *See bassinet day.*

average daily patient load—inpatient (ADPL-IP) – The average number of inpatients, excluding live births, in the hospital receiving care each day during a reported period; includes patients admitted and discharged on the same day. Calculated by dividing the number of inpatient bed days during the period by the total number of days in the report period.

average daily patient load—total (ADPL-TOT) – The average number of inpatients, including live births, in the hospital receiving care each day during a reported period; includes patients admitted and discharged on the same day, but excludes newborns. Calculated by dividing the sum of occupied bed days during the period by the total number of days in the report period.

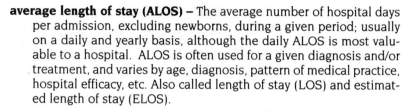

average length of stay (ALOS) – The average number of hospital days per admission, excluding newborns, during a given period; usually on a daily and yearly basis, although the daily ALOS is most valuable to a hospital. ALOS is often used for a given diagnosis and/or treatment, and varies by age, diagnosis, pattern of medical practice, hospital efficacy, etc. Also called length of stay (LOS) and estimated length of stay (ELOS).

average payment rate (APR) – The maximum amount that the Health Care Financing Administration (HCFA) will pay to an HMO or competitive medical plan (CMP) for Medicare services provided under a risk contract, weighted by age, sex and acuity.

average wholesale price (AWP) – The average cost for a pharmaceutical charged to pharmacy providers by pharmaceutical wholesaler suppliers.

avoidable hospital condition – Medical diagnosis for which hospitalization could have been avoided if ambulatory care had been provided in a timely and efficient manner.

B

bad debts – Accounts receivable that are considered uncollectable. In health care, this does not include charity write-offs associated with indigent (needy) care.

balance billing – The practice of billing a patient for the fee amount remaining after insurer payment and co-payment have been made. Under Medicare, the excess amount cannot be more than 15 percent above the approved charge.

Balanced Budget Act of 1997 (BBA) – A law that provided for several changes in health care including the establishment of medical savings accounts (MSA), the prospective payment system (PPS) for outpatient procedures (APCs or ambulatory patient classifications), and provider sponsored organizations (PSO). *See medical savings accounts, ambulatory patient classifications and provider sponsored organizations.*

base capitation – A specified amount per member per month (PMPM) to cover health care cost; usually excludes pharmacy and administrative costs as well as optional coverages such as mental health and substance abuse services.

base year costs – A Medicare term defined as the amount a hospital actually spent to render care in a previous time period. Depending on the hospital's Medicare cost reporting period, the base year was the fiscal year ending on or after September 30, 1982 and before September 30, 1983 for hospitals in operation at that time.

basic and major medical program – A program that combines basic "first-dollar" benefits with major medical-type benefits. First-dollar refers to insurance coverage that has no front-end deductible and coverage begins with the first dollar of expense incurred by the patient, for any covered benefit.

basic benefits – A set of "basic health services" specified in the member's certificate, plus services that are required under applicable federal and state laws and regulations.

basic coverage – Blue Cross and Blue Shield coverage exclusive of major medical. Basic coverage (Blue Cross and Blue Shield) will make payment first on a claim. As applied to Medicare beneficiaries, basic coverage would be Medicare Part A and/or Part B exclusive of any supplemental coverage.

B

basic health services
1. Benefits that all federally qualified HMOs must offer, defined under Subpart A, 110.102 of the Federal HMO Regulations.
2. The minimum supply of health services that should be generally available to assure adequate health care for a population. There is still some question between state and federal regulators and health insurance companies as to what constitutes an appropriate minimum set of services and how to assure their availability.

basic life insurance – A policy that provides a benefit when a person dies. The amount for which the person is insured is paid to the beneficiary designated on the policy if the covered person dies while still insured.

basic medical benefits – *See basic benefits.*

bassinet day – A day in which a live birth at the reporting facility occupied a bassinet in the newborn nursery at the time the census was taken. The stay must be continuous since birth, and is not dependent on the status of the mother.

batch balancing – A comparison of the number of items or documents that have been processed against a control total that has been predetermined. For example, a health insurance company issues 225 claims checks, which is batch balanced against 225 claims.

batch – A collection of charges and/or payments in a health insurance company's computer system. Most of these systems offer an on-line interactive system where all data entry immediately updates each account. Batches are employed for controlling data entry and providing an audit trail.

batch number – A designated number assigned to each data entry clerk for identification purposes when completing group or subscriber maintenance on all computer systems.

batch processing – A technique in which similar data or transactions are collected over a period of time and aggregated for sequential processing as a group during a machine run. Batch processing computer systems generally do not require immediate updating of files; data is gathered up to a cutoff time and then processed. The user receives the output after a period usually measured in hours or days.

BBA – *See Balance Budget Act of 1997.*

BCBSA – *See Blue Cross and Blue Shield Association.*

B

bed – Literally a bed in a hospital or other inpatient health facility. Beds are often used as a measure of capacity (hospital sizes are compared by their number of beds). Licenses and certificates-of-need (CON) may be granted for specific numbers or types of beds; e.g., surgical, pediatric, obstetric or extended care.

bed, available – A fully functioning bed that is available to a patient.

bed capacity – The number of beds that a hospital can accommodate.

bed capacity, expanded – The amount of space available for patient beds as measured by the number of beds that can be used in hospital units designed specifically for patients.

bed days/1000 – *See bed days per 1000.*

bed days per 1000 – The number of inpatient days per 1000 members of a defined population. Also called bed days/1000. *See admissions/1000.*

bed day, inpatient – A day spent by an adult or pediatric patient in a bed available for surgery patients or for standard inpatient admissions, at the census-taking hour, normally midnight, excluding bassinet days. It includes patients admitted and discharged on the same day, such as for same-day surgery.

bed, occupied by transient patient – A bed assigned as of midnight to a patient who is being moved between medical treatment facilities and who stops over while en route to his/her final destination.

bed, operating – *See operating bed.*

bed, set up – A bed that is ready in all respects for the care of a patient, except for the availability of staff. In other words, space, equipment, medical materiel, and ancillary and support services have been provided but the bed is not staffed to operate under normal circumstances.

beds, licensed – The number of beds that a hospital is licensed, certified, or otherwise authorized and has the capability to operate. Licensed beds means that space, equipment, medical materiel, and ancillary and support services have been provided, but the required staff is not necessarily available. Licensed beds equal the sum of operating beds and set up beds.

behavior health care – Assessment and treatment of mental and/or psychoactive substance abuse disorders. Also called behavioral health care.

benchmarking – The identification of best practices in the health care industry or another industry that exemplifies superior performance.

beneficial occupancy date (BOD) – The date on which a health care facility is available to serve the mission for which it was constructed.

beneficiary – A person who is entitled and eligible as either a subscriber or a dependent to receive benefits from a health insurance plan in accordance with a contract. Usually includes both the individual who has contracted for benefits and his/her eligible dependents. Also called eligible, enrollee or member.

beneficiary of benefits – *See beneficiary.*

benefit –
1. The care and services a payer will approve for payment under the provisions of a health insurance policy.
2. The actual amount of money a payer will pay for care and services.

benefit days –
1. The number of days for which a health insurance company will make payment within a benefit period.
2. The number of days for which the Medicare program will make payment for covered services on behalf of an entitled individual.

With the exception of lifetime reserve days, benefits are renewed with the start of each new benefit period.

benefit exhausted date – A Medicare term referring to the date on which the beneficiary has utilized his maximum benefits for the current benefit period. This only applies when the patient refuses to use or has exhausted his lifetime reserve days. Medicare provides a lifetime reserve of 60 days for payment of benefits beyond the normal limit. *See lifetime reserve days.*

benefit levels – The limitations or extent of benefits a person is entitled to receive based on his or her health insurance policy. In workers' compensation, benefit levels for injured workers are set by state law.

benefit limitations – Any provision, other than an exclusion, which restricts coverage regardless of medical necessity. Benefit limitations are explained in a health plan's explanation of coverage. *See explanation of coverage* (EOC).

B

benefit maximum – The maximum dollar amount that an insurance company or managed care company will cover for specific services.

benefit package – The list of covered services a health insurance plan or government agency offers to a group or individual. Benefit packages vary considerably. In addition to basic physician or hospital services, some health insurers cover prescriptions, vision care, chiropractic care, acupuncture, dental, alternative therapies, skilled nursing, assisted living care and even home nursing care.

Over time, employers and governments have shifted from a philosophy of offering a broad benefit package to making a "defined contribution" toward health coverage, although the beneficiary may opt to pay personally to receive a richer package of benefits. Sometimes called health benefits package, benefit plan, benefits and approved services.

benefit payment schedule – A listing of amounts an insurance plan will pay for covered health care services.

benefit period – The time period for which a person is eligible for covered benefits under a health insurance policy. The availability of certain benefits may be limited over a specified time period. For example, one physical examination within a one-year period. While the benefit period is usually defined by a set unit of time, benefits may also be tied to a condition or episode of illness.

benefit plan – *See benefit package.*

benefit products – Sometimes used by health insurance and managed care companies to refer to their health plans. Also used as a synonym for benefits.

benefits – Specific areas of a health plan's coverage (e.g., outpatient visits, hospitalization, etc.) that make up the range of medical services a health plan markets to its members and to which its members are entitled. The contractual agreement, specified in an evidence of coverage, indicates covered services provided by insurers to members. However, the fact that care is a membership benefit does not necessarily mean that charges for such care will be paid by the health plan either in full or in part. It depends upon the specifics of the evidence of coverage.

benefit year – A 12-month period that an employee group uses to administer its benefits program. The majority of employers use a benefit year from January through December. A benefit year does not always coincide with a group's fiscal year. *See benefit period.*

B

billing and accounts receivable (BAR) – Those automated functions which address the processes of billing and accounts receivable.

billing area – A tool some departments/divisions use to determine their clinical charges, payments and accounts receivables on a monthly basis. (For instance, plastic surgery, general surgery, and ENT are possible examples of billing areas.)

billed-at-home – *See direct pay*. Also called billed direct.

billed claims – Fees submitted by a health care provider for services rendered to a covered person.

bill cycle – Represents the day of the month on which certain groups are scheduled to be billed. There are 30 bill-cycle days per month including weekends and holidays.

bill frequency – Represents the regularity at which a subscriber or group is billed; usually monthly, quarterly or annually.

billed direct – *See direct pay*. Also called billed-at-home.

billing – A statement of dues or administrative charges.

billing address – The address to which billing is sent.

billing and service specialist – A clerk assigned to a group who handles collection of dues and charges, reconciliation and all subscriber maintenance, including correspondence.

birthday rule – In order to determine coordination of benefits (COB) where there is more than one insurance company covering the patient, the primary paying policy is the one taken out by the policyholder who has the birthday occurring earliest in the calendar year. If the birthdays of the policyholders occur on the same day, the policy that has been in effect the longest is considered primary. Year of birth does not enter into the birthday rule.

blanket coverage – Benefits under a family subscriber contract to dependents whose names and ages are not listed on the application form.

blanket medical expense – A provision (usually included as an added feature of a policy primarily providing some other type of coverage, such as loss of income insurance) which entitles the insured to collect up to a stated maximum established in the policy, for all hospital and medical expenses incurred, without limitations on individual types of medical expenses.

Blue Cross – Originally, a hospital insurance plan which provides ben-

B

efits covering specified hospital-related services and pays member hospitals directly for services rendered. *See Blue Cross/Blue Shield.*

Blue Cross/Blue Shield – General health insurance plans, affiliated through the Blue Cross Association, which include a large number of nonprofit and a few for-profit organizations that contract with hospitals, physicians and other health care providers to provide payment for health care services to their subscribers. Historically Blue Cross contracts have been with hospitals, and Blue Shield contracts with physicians.

Blue Cross and Blue Shield Association (BCBSA) – The national non-profit organization to which the Blue Cross and Blue Shield plans voluntarily belong. BCBSA administers programs of licensure and approval for Blue Cross and Blue Shield Plans, provides specific services related to the writing and administering of health care benefits across the country, and represents the Blue Cross and Blue Shield Plans in national affairs. Headquartered in Chicago, Illinois, BCBSA establishes administrative and fiscal standards that a local organization must meet in order to qualify as a Blue Cross and Blue Shield Plan.

Blue Cross and Blue Shield Board of Trustees – Governing bodies of Blue Cross and Blue Shield plans; members are elected to office from various sectors of business, government, and general publics. Also called board of directors.

Blue Cross logo – The registered symbol (a blue Greek cross with the figure of a man in the heart of the cross) and the words Blue Cross used to identify all Blue Cross plans.

Blue Cross plan – A not-for-profit corporation which administers a pre-payment program in a specific geographical service or plan area.

Blue Major – *See major medical.*

Blue Shield – Originally, a medical service insurance plan which provides benefits covering specified physician rendered services and pays either the physician or patient. *See Blue Cross/Blue Shield.*

Blue Shield logo – The registered symbol containing the caduceus (Greek healing symbol) impressed on a shield (protection). The Buffalo, New York, plan created the logo in 1939 based on the U.S. Army Medical Corps insignia.

Blue Shield plan – A not-for-profit corporation sponsored and/or approved by a medical society to administer a voluntary prepayment medical/surgical program in a specific service or plan area and operating under the membership standards of BCBSA.

B

board-certified – Physicians or other health professionals who have passed an examination given by a medical specialty board and have been certified by that board as a specialist in that area. Also called boarded or diplomate.

board certification – An official designation given by a recognized specialty board that a physician has met all requirements established for that specialty. Board certification is not legally required to practice a given specialty. Physicians who meet all criteria to apply for board certification but who do not have certification are sometimes called "board eligible".

board eligible – A physician who is eligible to take the specialty board examination by virtue of being graduated from an approved medical school, completing a specific type and length of training, and practicing for a specified amount of time.

Many managed care organizations restrict referrals to physicians without certification. However, some HMOs and other health facilities accept board eligibility as equivalent to board certification.

Boren Amendment – An amendment to the Omnibus Budget Reconciliation Act (OBRA 80, Public Law 96-499), which repealed the requirement that states follow Medicare principles in reimbursing hospitals, nursing facilities and ICFs/MR (intermediate care facility for mentally retarded persons) under the Medicaid program. The Boren Amendment substituted language which required states to develop payment rates which were "reasonable and adequate" to meet the costs of "efficiently and economically operated" providers. The amendment was intended to give states new flexibility, but it has also increased the number of successful lawsuits by providers and thus has contributed to the rising cost of Medicaid-funded institutional care. *See Omnibus Budget Reconciliation Act.*

brand name – The registered trademark given to a specific product by its manufacturer. Also known as trade name.

breach of confidentiality – Unauthorized release of confidential patient information to a third party.

break-even point – The membership level at which total revenues and total costs are equal and therefore produces neither a net gain nor loss from operations.

break-in-service – A defined term under ERISA (Employee Retirement Income Security Act) that signifies that an interruption in continuity of service has occurred. When an employee earns fewer than a

B

certain amount of hours of service in a computation period, a one-year break-in-service may occur and the plan may require that the employee re-establish a year of service in order to resume participation in the plan. *See Employee Retirement Income Security Act.*

broker – An insurance representative, licensed by the state, who places business with a variety of insurance companies. A broker represents the buyer of insurance rather than the companies, but is paid commissions by the companies. The broker may also render other services incidental to those functions. By law, the broker may also be an agent of the insurer for certain purposes such as delivery of the policy or collection of the premium.

BUBBA – The colloquial pronunciation of the BBA (Balanced Budget Act of 1997).

bundled billing – The setting of an exclusive package price or global fee for all the medical services required for a specific procedure, such as maternity care, coronary artery bypass graft or kidney transplant. Bundled billing usually includes both professional and institutional services.

bundled rate – *See flat fee-per-case.*

bundling – *See bundled billing.*

business coalition – A cooperative formed when several employers in a community join together to purchase health care at a lower cost for their employees.

C

CAA – Claims adjustment and analysis.

cafeteria plan – Benefit plans that are designed to give employees a degree of choice as to how their individual benefits are structured. Cafeteria plans generally provide core uniform benefits for all employees and allow individual employees to express some preferences. Also known as flexible benefit, flex plan or flexible compensation, these plans comply with Section 125 of the Internal Revenue Code.

CAHPS – *See consumer assessment of health plans survey.*

calendar year (CY) – A period of one year commencing January 1.

calendar year deductible – The most common form of deductible under major medical and comprehensive medical expense plans. Participants are permitted to accumulate covered expenses for the purpose of satisfying the deductible amount for the entire 12-month period.

call center – *See referral center.*

cap – Abbreviation for capitation.

capacity – The ability of a health care organization to provide necessary health services.

capitation (CAP) – A method of payment for health services in which the provider is paid a fixed, per member per month (PMPM) amount for each person served without regard to the frequency of utilization or nature of services provided. The provider agrees to be responsible for delivering or arranging all health services required by the patient, and is not reimbursed for services that exceed the allotted capitation amount (at risk). Capitation is characteristic of Health Maintenance Organizations (HMOs), and mostly for primary care services, although a few specialty capitation plans do exist. *See capitation rate and risk.*

capitation rate (cap rate) – A dollar amount established to cover the expected cost of services provided to a person. The cap rate is primarily applied to beneficiaries of group health plans and, more specifically, Health Maintenance Organization (HMO) services. Typically, a provider receives the per capita rate payment, usually on a per member per month (PMPM) basis, and is accountable for delivering or arranging for all health care services required by the

C

patient. Although cap rates are usually fixed, they can be adjusted for the age or gender of members based on actuarial (statistical) projections of health care utilization. *See actuarial.*

captive insurance company – An insurance company formed to underwrite (insure) the risks of its owners (e.g., a hospital system that either forms or buys its own insurance companies).

captured care – Percentage of a provider's care provided under exclusive managed care contracts and/or capitation arrangements.

cardiology – Branch of medicine dealing with the treatment and diagnosis of the heart and blood vessels.

care – Services, equipment, supplies and hospital accommodations provided or used for diagnosis or treatment of a condition.

care management – *See case management.*

care mapping – *See disease management.*

carrier – A commercial health insurer, a government agency, or a Blue Cross or Blue Shield Plan which underwrites or administers programs that pay for health services. Organizations that hold contracts with the Social Security Administration to handle medical claims under Part B of Medicare are also called carriers.

carrier replacement (CR) – A situation where a sole health insurance carrier replaces one or more other health insurance carriers on a specific group client. Carrier replacement allows consolidation of the group's experience and risk.

carryover or carry-over – A provision in health plans to avoid two deductibles applied to covered medical expenses when expenses are incurred toward the end of one calendar year and the sickness or injury continues into the next year.

carve-out –
1. A payer strategy to separately purchase a portion of the overall medical benefits from a specialty managed care organization. For example, a health plan may "carve out" behavioral health and contract with a specialty managed behavioral health company to provide these services to the health plan's members. Many health insurance companies use carve-out services either because they do not have the in-house expertise or costs are such that it would be more efficient to use an outside vendor. Other examples of carve-outs include vision and dental. Sometimes called single service plan (SSP).

C

2. A form of retiree medical coverage where the regular plan of benefits continues to apply to retirees, but plan benefits are reduced by the amount of allowances from Medicare.

case – A covered instance of illness or injury.

case managed – *See case management.*

case management – A process that identifies patients with specific health care needs, then plans and manages their health care to achieve the optimum outcome in the most cost-effective manner. Identified patients (members) are usually the chronically ill or otherwise impaired individual who may require long term and/or costly care. These patients are sometimes referred to as "case managed." The goal of case management is to coordinate the care so as to both improve continuity and quality of care, as well as lower costs of care.

Case management attempts to match the appropriate intensity of services with the patient's needs over time. It also helps to avoid unnecessary testing and care by preventing medical problems from escalating, and can often produce alternatives to institutional care that result in better patient outcomes as well as lower costs. The patient is assigned a case manager who may act as an assessor, facilitator, planner and advocate for the individual during the process. Case management is sometimes a carve-out. *See carve-out.*

case manager – A skilled professional (e.g., nurse, physician or social worker) who works with patients, providers and insurers to coordinate all services deemed necessary to provide the patient with a plan of medically necessary and appropriate health care.

case mix – A method of categorizing patients in a hospital or post acute facility using factors such as diagnosis, procedure, severity of illness, utilization of services, provider characteristics, method of payment, etc. Case mix helps measure a hospital's rate of admissions, capabilities and needs. This concept and how it is applied can vary by region or locale of the country.

case mix index – An index that shows the relative cost of treatment on an inpatient basis. Indexes are based on the average, which is set at 1.00. An index of 1.04 means that the facility's inpatients are 4% more costly than average. An index of .96 mean that the facility's inpatients are 4% less costly than average.

case rate – *See flat fee per case.*

C

case-rate capitation – Refers to reimbursement of specialists (e.g., orthopedists, urologists, oncologists, etc.) based on a referral or an episode of care. Also called contract capitation. *See specialist.*

cash indemnity benefits – Sums that are paid to an insured person for covered services and that require submission of a filed claim. The insured may assign such payments directly to providers of services such as hospitals or physicians. This is known as assignment of benefits. Payments may or may not fully reimburse the insured for costs incurred.

catastrophic case – Any medical condition where total cost of treatment, regardless of payment source, is expected to exceed an amount designated by the HMO contract with the medical group.

catastrophic health insurance – Health insurance which provides protection against the high cost of treating severe or lengthy illnesses or disabilities. In most cases, catastrophic health insurance policies cover medical expenses above an amount that is the responsibility of the insured, up to a maximum limit of liability. There is usually no maximum amount of coverage under these plans, but many include some coinsurance.

Catastrophic health insurance is less expensive than traditional indemnity insurance or managed care plans and, as such, is most attractive to the population that is younger, healthier and less concerned about "full" health insurance coverage. Often called major medical, catastrophic insurance and catastrophic plan.

catastrophic insurance – *See catastrophic health insurance.*

catastrophic plan – *See catastrophic health insurance.*

catchment area – The defined geographic area served by a hospital, clinic or health plan, determined by such factors as population distribution, accessibility and geographic boundaries. Studies of catchment areas are useful in determining potentially new health care services.

catchment area management – A concept where health services planning and resource budgeting are based on the beneficiary population.

categorical programs – Public health insurance programs designed to benefit a certain category of people; for example, Medicare for the elderly and some disabled individuals, and Medicaid for the indigent.

C

CCN – *See community care networks.*

CDC – Claims distribution center.

CDC – *See Centers for Disease Control and Prevention.*

CEE – Claims evaluation and entry.

census – In health insurance, refers to a statistical listing of enrollees in a group by age, sex, marital status, number of dependents, etc. In a hospital setting, refers to the patient population.

Centers for Disease Control and Prevention (CDC) – Located in Atlanta, Georgia, the CDC provides facilities and services for the investigation, prevention and control of diseases; supports quarantine and other activities to prevent introduction of communicable diseases from foreign countries; conducts research into the epidemiology, laboratory diagnosis, prevention and treatment of infectious and other controllable diseases at the community level; provides grants for work on venereal disease, immunization against infectious diseases, and disease control programs; and sets standards for laboratories.

centers of excellence (COE) – Hospitals and other health care facilities that specialize in treating specific illnesses, such as cancer, or performing specific treatments, such as organ transplants.

certificate – The legal document certifying the terms of membership and benefits to which a health plan member is entitled.

certificate membership benefit maximum(s) – The maximum total of payments that a health plan will make for certain types of care that a member may receive while the certificate is in effect.

certificate number – A number assigned to a membership for identification. Also called identification number.

certificate of authority (COA) – A certificate issued by a state government that licenses the operation of a Health Maintenance Organization (HMO).

certificate of coverage (COC) – The formal agreement between a subscriber and the health plan describing the benefits included in a carrier's plan. The COC is required by state law. Also called evidence of coverage (EOC), subscriber agreement, benefit plan and insurance policy.

certificate of insurance – A statement issued to a member of a group certifying that an insurance contract covering the member has been

C

written and contains a summary of the terms applicable to that member.

certificate of need (CON) – A certificate issued by a state agency that legally authorizes a health care institution to construct or modify a health care facility, change health services offered, or acquire expensive medical equipment. Before the CON is issued, the request is reviewed to ensure that the facility or service meets the need of those for whom it is intended. Federally qualified HMOs do not need to apply for CONs.

certification – The process by which an agency or association evaluates and recognizes a person who meets predetermined standards. "Certification" is usually applied to individuals and "accreditation" to institutions.

certification and recertification of service need – Refers to the requirement that a physician attest to the need for hospitalization and continued stay, usually upon admission and at stated intervals thereafter.

certified health consultant (CHC) – An individual who has successfully completed the CHC program demonstrating a broad knowledge of the field of health care financing. CHCs are generally recognized as expert consultants to purchasers of employee benefit packages and administrators of employee health care benefit programs. *See certified health consultant program.*

certified health consultant program – A series of comprehensive examinations in the health care financing process that test an individual's knowledge of health care economics, pricing, underwriting, financing mechanisms, marketing and selling skills. In addition to passing each of these examinations, the certification process requires that the candidate successfully complete two weeks of residency training (The National Marketing Development Institute - Parts I and III). The program was developed by the Blue Cross Blue Shield Association in 1978.

certified nurse-midwife (CNM) – An individual educated in the two disciplines of nursing and midwifery who possesses evidence of certification according to the requirements of the American College of Nurse Midwifery (ACNM). The CNM has advanced training and education in nursing and maternity care.

certified registered nurse anesthetist (CRNA) – A registered nurse who has been trained, certified and who specializes in the administration of anesthetics during surgical procedures. Nurse anes-

C

thetist education builds on prior nursing experience with a curriculum that incorporates anatomy, physiology, pathophysiology, chemistry, physics, biochemistry, and pharmacology as they relate to anesthesia. Graduates of nurse anesthetist programs must pass the national certification exam to become CRNAs.

CHAMPUS – See *Civilian Health and Medical Program of the Uniformed Services.*

CHAMPVA – See *Civilian Health and Medical Program of the Veterans Administration.*

channeling – The efforts and ability to direct patients to particular providers or hospitals. For example, health plans often attempt to "channel" patients to providers in the plan's network rather than outside of the network. *See network.*

charge – The dollar amount charged for a service or procedure by a provider.

charge-based reimbursement – Payments to institutional providers for the actual incurred costs of covered services plus reimbursement for bad debts, cost of charity cases, and a profit.

charge document – The form generated when a patient receives services containing patient demographics, services rendered (CPT) codes, diagnosis (ICD-9 and ICD-10) codes and charges for each service. Also called an encounter form.

charge entry – Process in which charges are entered into the billing and collection system.

charges – Prices assigned to units of medical service, such as a visit to a physician or a day in a hospital. Charges for services may not be related to the actual costs of providing the services, and the methods by which charges are related to costs vary substantially from service to service and institution to institution. Charges for one service provided by an institution are often used to subsidize the costs of other services. Similarly, charges to one group of patients may also be used to subsidize the cost of providing services to other groups.

CHC – See *certified health consultant* or *community health center.*

cherry picking – The practice of enrolling only healthy individuals and not accepting individuals with existing health problems.

child conversion code – The code that indicates how long a dependent child is covered under family membership (e.g., end of calendar year of limiting age, birth date, etc.).

C

CHIN – *See community health information network.*

chiropodist – A podiatrist. *See Doctor of Podiatric Medicine* (DPM).

chiropractic services – A system of mechanical therapeutics based on the principles that the nervous system largely determines the state of health and that disease results from abnormal nerve function conformity.

chiropractor – A practitioner of chiropractic services (mechanical therapeutics) consisting primarily of the manipulation of parts of the body, especially the spinal column. Some chiropractors also use physiotherapy, nutritional supplements and other therapeutic modalities. Chiropractors are licensed by all states. *See chiropractic services.* Also called Doctor of Chiropractic (DC).

chronic care – Long-term care of individuals with long-standing, persistent diseases or conditions. Chronic care often includes the promotion of self-care to help the individual prevent the loss of function.

chronic care network (CCN) – A network of health care providers who provide service to patients with chronic (long term) conditions. The network can be composed of hospitals, physicians, pharmacists, physical therapists, etc.

chronic disease – A disease which has one or more of the following characteristics: is permanent, leaves residual disability, is caused by non-reversible pathological alternation, requires special training of the patient for rehabilitation, or may be expected to require a long period of observation or care.

churning – The practice of a provider seeing a patient more often than is medically necessary, primarily to increase revenue through an increased number of services. In health insurance, churning refers to the continual replacement of lost customers with new ones.

CIS – *See clinical information systems.*

Civilian Health and Medical Program of the Uniformed Services (CHAMPUS) – A program administered by the Department of Defense, without premium but with cost-sharing provisions, that pays for care delivered by civilian health providers to retired members and dependents of active and retired members of the seven uniformed services of the U.S. (Army, Navy, Air force, Marines, Coast Guard, Air National Guard, National Guard).

C

Civilian Health and Medical Program of the Veterans Administration (CHAMPVA) – A program administered by the Department of Defense for the Veterans Administration, without premium but with cost-sharing provisions, that pays for health care provided by civilian providers to dependents of totally disabled veterans who are eligible for retirement pay from a uniformed service.

claim – A notification and request for payment to an insurance or managed care company from either a provider or covered person that a patient received medical services or supplies. The term "claim" generally refers to the liability for health care services received by covered persons, and is the actual notification that begins the processing for payment.

claim denial – The formal refusal of a health plan to reimburse for a medical procedure following a claims review. The denial typically states the reason for the refusal to reimburse.

claim form – Itemization of activity, either on paper or on computer tape, that is sent to an insurance company.

claim number – Number assigned and used by the claims administrator to identify a claim record and its history.

claims administrative expense (CAE) – Costs arising directly from the processing or investigation of claims.

claims administrator – The organization responsible for processing of claims and associated services for a health plan.

claims review – The method by which a health plan reviews an enrollee's medical claims prior to reimbursement. The claims review includes determining the eligibility of the enrollee and the provider, ensuring that the benefit is not payable under another policy, validating the necessity of the care, and making sure the cost of the service is not excessive.

claim status – Classification used for designating whether or not a given claim will be paid, such as "approved," "denied" or "pending."

claims, unreported – *See incurred but not reported.*

class of risk – A body of subscribers ranked together as having common characteristics and subject to an equal chance of loss; for instance, a group of male smokers over the age of 50.

client – A person who is enrolled in the Medicaid program and eligible to receive services funded through Medicaid. *See also recipient.*

C

clinic – A facility for the provision of preventive, diagnostic and treatment services to outpatients. The term "clinic" has been used in diverse ways, including describing facilities that have physician offices, are equipped with beds, serve poor or public patients, or practice medical education.

clinical data repository – The part of a computer-based patient record (CPR) which stores clinical data from a variety of supplemental treatment and intervention systems. The data can be used for practice guidelines, outcomes management and clinical research. Sometimes referred to as a data warehouse.

clinical decision support – The capability of a computer system to provide data to health care providers and clinicians in response to "flags" based on embedded, provider-created rules. An example would be a system that would alert case managers that a patient's eligibility for a certain service is about to be exhausted. Clinical decision support is a crucial functional requirement to support clinical or critical pathways.

clinical information systems (CIS) – A computer system that maintains a database based on actual patient information on care and treatment. The CIS is often used for decision support. *See clinical decision support.*

clinical pathways – A "map" of preferred treatment/intervention activities. Clinical pathways outline the types of information needed by providers to make decisions, the timelines for applying that information, and what action needs to be taken by whom. They also provide a way to monitor care "in real time." These pathways are developed by clinicians for specific diseases or events. Proactive providers work to develop these pathways for the majority of their interventions and develop the software capacity to distribute and store this information. Also called critical pathways.

clinical privileges – Permission to provide medical, dental and other patient care services in the granting institution (e.g., hospital), within defined limits, based on the individual's education, professional license, experience, competence, ability, health and judgment.

clinical protocols – Guidelines developed by medical professionals for treating specific injuries and conditions, and to evaluating the appropriateness of specific procedures.

clinical psychologists – A health professional specializing in the evaluation and treatment of mental and behavioral disorders. Clinical psychologists are licensed by most states for independent profes-

C

sional practice and their services are reimbursed by many health insurance programs. They do not treat physical causes of mental illness with drugs or other medical or surgical measures since they are not licensed to practice medicine.

clinical service organization (CSO) – An organization created by academic medical centers to integrate the activities of the medical school, faculty practice plan and hospital to negotiate with managed care plans.

clinician – A medical or dental practitioner having admitting privileges and primary responsibility for care of inpatients.

clinic without walls – *See group without walls* (GWW).

closed access – A type of health plan that requires covered persons to receive care from providers within the plan's coverage and to coordinate their care through a primary care physician serving as the patient's initial contact and referral source; otherwise known as "gatekeeper." Except for emergencies, the patient may only be referred to and treated by providers within the plan.

closed formulary – A listing of drugs that a health plan limits drug prescribers to choose from and its pharmacy members to dispense. In a closed formulary, a health plan will not reimburse pharmacists or patients for drugs that are not on the formulary. Also called a select or mandatory formulary.

closed panel – An insurance plan that allows members to receive non-emergency health services only through a specific limited number of providers or facilities. Closed panel usually refers to a group or staff model HMO. The problem with a closed panel for members is that their preferred physician or facility may not be in the panel.

CMP – *See competitive medical plan.*

coalition – An association of health care plan sponsors who pool their resources to negotiate with insurers or other health care payers and providers.

COA – *See certificate of authority.*

COB – *See coordination of benefits.*

COBRA – *See Consolidated Omnibus Budget Reconciliation Act.*

COC – *See certificate of coverage.*

coinsurance – The percentage of eligible expenses that patients must pay for certain care each year until they reach their coinsurance

C

maximum. This is in addition to a deductible, and generally runs in the 10 to 20 percent range. For example, a typical 80/20 coinsurance plan means 80% of health care expenses is paid by the company and 20% is paid by the insured member.

Coinsurance and deductibles are most commonly found in indemnity, fee-for-service and PPO plans. Coinsurance should not be confused with cooperative payment or copayment.

coinsurance maximum – The amount that a patient must pay in eligible coinsurance expenses each year before a health plan will cover 100% of eligible expenses for the remainder of the year.

collections per 1000 – An indicator calculated by taking the total collections for services received by a specific group, (e.g., employer group) for a specific period of time, dividing it by the average number of covered members or lives in that group during that period, and multiplying the result by 1000.

This indicator may be calculated in aggregate or by modality of treatment (e.g., inpatient, partial hospitalization and outpatient). Collections per 1000 is also a measure used to evaluate utilization management performance. Proactive providers should have either developed or be developing the capacity to measure their performance along such dimensions.

commercial carrier – A private insurance company (usually for-profit) that provides health care benefits to a group or individual.

commercial plan – Refers to the benefit package an insurance company/HMO/PPO offers to employers, as opposed to a senior plan which is offered to Medicare beneficiaries.

commission on professional and hospital activities (CPHA) – A nonprofit, non-government organization based in Ann Arbor, Michigan, established in 1965 which collects, processes and distributes data on hospital use for management, evaluation and research purposes. The system abstracts and classifies information in a computer-accessible data library.

commissions – The fees of a salesman, broker, agent, etc.

community-based waiver – *See Section* 1915.

community care network (CCN) – One name for what is known as accountable health plans. Community care networks (CCN) tend to be community-based and non-profit. *See accountable health plans.*

C

community health center (CHC) – Health centers that provide care to the indigent within communities.

community health information network (CHIN) – An integrated set of computer and telecommunication capabilities that permit multiple providers, payers, employers and related health care entities within a geographic area to share and communicate client, clinical and payment information. Also known as community health management information system.

community-oriented primary care (COPC) – Combines the elements of good primary care delivery with a community population-based approach to identifying and addressing health problems in the community.

community rating – A method for setting health insurance rates based on the average cost of providing health services to all people in a specific geographic area. Rates are not dependent on individual claim experience or the experience of any group. The result is that plan subscribers pay the same rate for the same level of benefits regardless of their age, sex or health status.

Community rating spreads the costs of health care evenly over all subscribers rather than charging the sick more than the healthy for coverage. Federally qualified HMOs are required to use community rating. Under the laws of many states, other HMOs might be required to use community rating, but may also be permitted to factor in differences for age, sex, contract size or industry. Sometimes called pooled rate. Compare to experience rating.

Community rating can effectively lower premiums for health plans with adverse selection (members who are prone to higher than average utilization), but may also raise rates for health plans that have young or healthy people who will not utilize most benefits. *See also adjusted community rating.*

community rating by class (CRC) – *See adjusted community rating.*

comorbidity – Coexisting medical conditions that together could complicate a patient's health status and treatment procedures. Comorbidity makes it more difficult to treat each condition separately and may increase hospital length of stay. Sometimes referred to as comorbidity condition.

comparability – In general, comparability means that each state must ensure that the same Medicaid benefits are available to all people who are eligible. Exceptions include: 1) benefits approved under

C

Medicaid waiver programs for special sub-populations of Medicaid eligibles, and 2) benefits available to children through EPSDT (Early and Periodic Screening, Diagnosis, and Treatment), which may not be available to adults.

compendium – A collection of information about drugs. Under the Federal Food, Drug, and Cosmetic Act, standards for strength, quality, and purity of drugs are those which are set forth in one of the three official compendia: the *United States Pharmacopea*, the *Homeopathic Pharmacopea of the United States*, the *National Formulary*, or any supplement to any of them.

Competitive Medical Plan (CMP) – A designation by the federal government that enables a health plan to be eligible for Medicare risk contracts, without qualifying as an HMO. The CMP designation requirements are less restrictive than an HMO. The CMP status was established by TEFRA (Tax Equity and Fiscal Responsibility Act).

complementary programs – Special programs offered to participants in Medicare Parts A and B to supplement the medical coverage.

complete care organization (CCO) – Hospitals and providers working cooperatively to provide care within a community.

completion factor – Monthly factor used to adjust incurred and paid claims to expected incurred claims.

complication – A medical condition that develops during a patient's course of treatment that alters the course of the illness or treatment, and is expected to increase the length of stay by at least one day.

composite rate – One premium rate applied to all members in a group regardless of the number of their dependents. Composite rate is also used to describe the average unit cost per employee covered.

comprehensive healthcare clinic (CHCC) – A facility planned and constructed to provide comprehensive ambulatory care services with limited holding bed capability.

comprehensive health planning – Health planning which encompasses all factors and programs which impact on people's health.

comprehensive major medical (CMM) – Health care coverage that combines basic hospital, basic medical/surgical and supplemental major medical benefits into one plan with cost sharing features such as deductible and coinsurance. It is a complete package of health care services and benefits generally characterized by a low

C

deductible and high maximum benefits, including prevention, early detection and early treatment of conditions. Sometimes known as a comprehensive program, comprehensive medical care and comprehensive major medical insurance.

comprehensive medical care – See *comprehensive major medical.*

comprehensive program – See *comprehensive major medical.*

computer-based patient record (CPR) – A term for the process of replacing the traditional paper-based patient medical chart through automated electronic means. In other words, collecting patient-specific information from various treatment systems and storing it within a computer database for individual as well as aggregate patient purposes. Also called electronic medical record, online medical record and paperless patient chart. See *formatting and protocol standards.*

CON – See *certificate of need.*

concurrent care – See *concurrent medical care.*

concurrent medical care – A situation that occurs when two or more doctors are providing inpatient hospital care to the same patient. Usually, they are treating separate and unrelated conditions, but it is possible they are providing care for the same diagnosis on the same day. Also called concurrent care.

concurrent review – The process by which the course of a patient's treatment is reviewed for appropriateness and by which continued stays at a hospital are verified for medical necessity and level of care. This usually occurs for inpatient, residential and partial hospitalization treatment, but is becoming more frequent for outpatient as well. The review is typically done at the time services are being rendered by a health care professional other than the one providing the care. See *medical necessity.*

condition – Defined as any illness, disease, bodily injury, pregnancy, bodily defect or abnormality, mental illness, alcoholism, drug addiction or chemical dependency.

confinement – See *hospital confinement.*

Consolidated Omnibus Budget Reconciliation Act of 1985 (COBRA) – A federal law that, among other things, requires employers to offer continued health insurance coverage to certain employees and their beneficiaries whose group health insurance coverage has been terminated. The specific qualified events provided for in the law

C

include: termination for non-misconduct acts, reduction in employment hours, death of employee, divorce, legal separation, entitlement to Medicare benefits or dependent child reaching maximum age for coverage.

The law does not affect employers with fewer than 20 employees, plans for federal employees, church plans or association groups (except for employers with 20 or more employees within the association).

consolidation – Refers to a concentration of control by a few health care organizations over other existing health care organizations by unifying their facilities. Hospital mergers, acquisitions, alliances, and the formation of contractual networks are examples of consolidation. Related to integration. *See integration.*

consultant – An expert in a specific medical, dental or other health services field who provides specialized professional advice or services upon request.

consultation – In medical or dental practice, the act of requesting advice from another provider, usually a specialist, regarding the diagnosis and/or treatment of a patient. The consultant usually reviews the history, examines the patient, and then provides his/her written or oral opinion to the requesting practitioner.

consulting nurse – A registered nurse (RN) who is trained to assess health problems over the phone. The nurse can advise patients regarding symptoms, possible home care, and when and where to seek medical care.

consulting physician – A physician called upon to examine a patient and/or the patient's record to advise the attending physician on treatment.

consumer assessment of health plans survey (CAHPS) – A yearly nationwide survey that reports information on Medicare beneficiaries' experiences and satisfaction with receiving care in managed care plans. The survey is based on a database using a HEDIS subset and 33 Medicare-related measures.

contact lenses – Ophthalmic corrective lenses, either glass or plastic, ground or molded. They must be prescribed by a physician or optometrist to be directly fitted to the eye.

contingency fees – Fees based or conditioned on future occurrences or conclusions, or on the results of services to be performed. Contingency fees are used by lawyers representing patients as

C

plaintiffs in malpractice cases and are usually a set percent of any settlement awarded the patient. If no settlement is awarded, the lawyer is not paid.

contingency reserve – A health plan's reserve fund allocated to meet the cost of unexpected occurrences

contingent beneficiary – Person(s) named to receive benefits if the primary beneficiary is not alive.

continued stay review – A review, usually conducted by a hospital or health plan, to determine if the current place of service is still the most appropriate to provide the level of care required by the patient.

continuing education – Education beyond initial professional preparation that is relevant to the type of patient care delivered within a health care organization and provides current knowledge relevant to an individual's field of health care practice. Also called continuing medical education.

continuity of care – Health care provided on a continuous basis beginning with the patient's initial contact with a primary care physician and following the patient through all episodes. Essentially, care that is uninterrupted.

continuous care – Nursing care provided on a continuous basis up to 24-hours-a-day during a period of crisis as necessary to maintain an individual at home. A period of crisis is a period when the member requires continuous care to relieve or manage acute medical symptoms, including emotional support during the last stage of the patient's illness.

continuous coverage – Transferring from one covered health plan group to another with no break in coverage, or from one form of membership to another; such as from dependent to subscriber with acquiring a different subscriber identification number.

continuous home care day – A day on which an individual who has elected to receive hospice care is not in an inpatient facility and receives hospice care consisting predominantly of nursing care on a continuous basis at home. Home health aides or other home services may also be provided on a continuous basis. Continuous home care is only furnished during brief periods of crisis and only as necessary to maintain a terminally ill patient at home.

continuum of care – A range of medical, nursing treatments and social services in a variety of settings that provides services most appro-

C

priate to the level of care required. For example, the range of services from inpatient to stepped-down referrals to community support groups is a continuum of care.

Continuum of care is "one-stop shopping" that allows employers and managed care organizations to contract for a full range of services from a single provider, such as a hospital offering services ranging from nursery to a hospice. Providers can pinpoint a niche market and sell that service to a contracting group or facility in order to find a place along the continuum of care.

continuous quality improvement (CQI) – The process of applying sophisticated techniques (e.g., decision support systems) to identify problems in the delivery of health care services, developing solutions and constantly monitoring those solutions for improvement. CQI is intended to encourage appropriate and necessary care, as well as accountability for cost and quality. Sometimes called total quality management (TQM).

contract – In legal terms, a contract is an agreement between two or more parties to perform specific services or duties in return for monetary or other consideration. In managed care terms, a contract is a legal agreement between a health plan and a subscribing group or individual that specifies rates, eligibility limitations, benefit descriptions, performance covenants and other pertinent conditions.

The contract is usually limited to a 12-month period and is subject to renewal thereafter. Contracts are not required by statute or regulation, so less formal agreements can be made.

contract capitation – *See case rate capitation.*

contract mix – The distribution of the types of enrollees in a health plan, usually classified by dependency. That is, the number or percentage of singles, subscriber and spouse, subscriber and children, etc. Contract mix is used to determine average contract size.

contract group – *See enrolled group.*

contract month – One month within a contract period. The term "contract month" is primarily used by insurance companies and managed care organizations to describe utilization or market share expressed in terms of the number of subscriber contracts per month.

contract number – A numerical designation assigned by a health plan to each employer or individual plan that helps identify the benefits

C

of the specific health care plan.

contract provider – Any provider that has a contractual arrangement with a health insurance plan to provide services to the plan's members. Providers include physicians, dentists, pharmacists, hospitals, ambulatory surgical centers, home health care agencies, skilled nursing facilities, and extended care facilities.

contract type – Identifies the set of member relationships under which a health plan subscriber can enroll. *See coverage type.*

contract year – A period of 12 consecutive months, beginning with the beginning date of coverage. The 12-month period may not always coincide with a calendar year.

contracting hospital – A hospital that has contracted with a health plan to provide certain hospital services to members.

contractual allowance – A contract between a provider and a health plan to provide services for a predetermined fee. Most often used when describing a discounted fee arrangement.

contribution requirements – The amount an employer is required to pay toward the cost of coverage for employees or employees and dependents. For example, an employer may be required to pay a minimum of 75% of the cost of an employee's coverage but nothing toward the cost of dependents, or at least 50% of the cost for both the employee and dependents.

contributory program – A group plan in which members and their employer share the cost of health insurance, normally through payroll deductions.

control plan – A Blue Cross Blue Shield term meaning the Blue Cross Blue Shield Plan which has the primary responsibility in administering a group that is served by more than one Blue Cross Blue Shield Plan. This situation only occurs when a health plan crosses into states covered by other Blue Cross Blue Shield plans.

controller – The officer in charge of the funds of a company or an organization.

convalescent care – Care rendered to patients who are ambulatory. Complexity of care requires limited therapeutic intervention and administration of oral medications performed by the patient. Patients are in the final stages of recovery and care emphasis is on physical reconditioning.

C

conventional group insurance – *See indemnity plan.*

conversion – *See conversion privilege.*

conversion clause – The privilege granted in a group insurance policy to convert to an individual insurance policy upon termination of group coverage.

conversion factor (CF) – The dollar amount used to multiply the relative value scale (RVS) of a procedure to arrive at the maximum allowable for that procedure. That is, the price to be paid to the provider for a given service equals the relative value of the service multiplied by the dollar amount of the conversion factor. For example, if a provider runs a blood sugar determination on a patient, the procedure might have a relative value (RVS) of 5.0, and the conversion factor might be $5.00. The "price" of the blood sugar determination would therefore be $25.00.

conversion members – Individuals who are no longer members of an employer group, but are still eligible to receive continuation of their benefits from health plans under COBRA (Consolidated Omnibus Reconciliation Act) regulations.

conversion plan – A plan that allows members to continue health care coverage under an individual plan when their group plan is canceled.

conversion privilege – A privilege granted in an insurance policy giving individuals the right to convert their group insurance to an individual policy without a medical examination upon termination of their group insurance.

cooperating provider – A licensed health care professional who has entered into a written agreement with a health plan to provide health care to the plan's members.

cooperative payments – *See copayment.*

coordinated care – Another term for managed care.

coordination of benefits (COB) – A process to coordinate the reimbursement of benefits when an individual is covered by two or more health plans. Coordination of benefits is usually written into an insurance policy or stipulated by state law, and eliminates overinsurance or duplication of benefits. The primary carrier provides its coverage first, with the secondary carrier providing any additional covered benefits. The payment from both carriers combined may not exceed 100% of the covered benefits for all medical expenses.

C

copay or co-pay – *See copayment.*

copayment or co-payment – A cost sharing arrangement in which a plan member (covered person) pays a specified charge for a specified service, such as $10 for an office visit. The member is usually responsible for payment at the time the health care is rendered. Typical co-payments are fixed or variable flat amounts for physician office visits, prescriptions or hospital services. The amount paid must be nominal to avoid becoming a barrier to care. It does not vary with the cost of the service, unlike co-insurance which is based on some percentage of cost. Also called co-pay or cooperative payments. *See also cost sharing, coinsurance and deductibles.*

COPC – *See community-oriented primary care.*

corporate practice of medicine – State laws prohibiting lay people, organizations and corporations from directly or indirectly practicing medicine. They are designed to ensure that those making decisions about the provision of medical services will not be subject to commercial exploitation.

cosmetic surgery – Any operation directed at improving appearance. In health insurance, cosmetic surgery is differentiated from reconstructive surgery. That is, most health insurance plans and programs do not cover cosmetic surgery unless it is the result of a catastrophic event or surgery that results in disfigurement of the individual; for example, radical mastectomy resulting in breast reconstruction (reconstructive surgery). Cosmetic surgery is also known as aesthetic surgery. *See reconstructive surgery.*

cost-based reimbursement – Payment of all "allowable" costs incurred in the provision of care, based on the terms of the contract under which care is furnished.

cost-benefit analysis – An analytic method in which a program's cost is compared to the program's benefits for a period of time, expressed in dollars, as an aid in determining the best investment of resources. For example, the cost of establishing an immunization service might be compared with the total cost of medical care and lost productivity, which will be eliminated as a result of more persons being immunized. Cost-benefit analysis can also be applied to specific medical tests and treatments.

cost containment – Activities that restrain the cost of medical care or reduce its escalation rate. Cost containment is attained by reducing administrative costs, controlling the utilization of health care services, limiting the demand for services, and managing other con-

C

ditions that contribute to higher than necessary costs. Some strategies utilized under cost containment include capitation, preventive care, wellness programs, and disease management. Cost containment is a major objective of managed care organizations.

cost contract – A TEFRA (Tax Equity and Fiscal Responsibility Act) contract payment methodology option by which HCFA pays for the delivery of health services to members based on the HMO's reasonable cost. The plan receives an interim amount derived from an estimated annual budget, which may be periodically adjusted during the course of the contract to reflect actual cost experience. The plan's expenses are audited at the end of the contract to determine the final rate the plan should have been paid.

cost effectiveness – Refers to the additional benefits that can be derived from doing something in relation to the additional costs that must be incurred. *See cost-benefit analysis and efficacy.*

cost-efficiency – *See cost effectiveness.*

cost outlier – A patient who is more costly to treat compared with other patients in a particular diagnosis-related group. A term that is often used in Medicare.

Cost Plus –
1. A health insurance funding mechanism where the carrier assumes no underwriting risk. The insured group pays the cost of the benefits (or incurred claims) plus administrative costs, plus a contribution to the carrier's contingency reserve.
2. A method of reimbursement for hospital stays where total operating costs and certain allowable capital costs are included in arriving at the per diem (per day) rate. When the amount of reimbursement from a payer becomes inadequate or when uncompensated services are rendered, providers resort to cost shifting by charging extra to those payers who do not exercise strict cost controls. Cost Plus has been the typical means for rendering uncompensated care to the uninsured.

cost plus reimbursement – A reimbursement method where providers are paid based on their actual costs plus a profit. Occurs under fee-for-service (FFS) plans.

cost reimbursement – A method of reimbursing providers based on their actual incurred costs.

cost sharing – Describes the provisions of a health insurance policy which require the insured or otherwise covered individuals to pay

C

some portion of their covered medical expenses. Cost sharing includes co-payments, coinsurance and deductibles, and, at times, may also occur when an insured pays a portion of the monthly premium for health care insurance.

Co-payments are flat fees that insured persons must pay for a particular unit of service, such as an office visit, emergency room visit, or the filling of a drug prescription. Coinsurance is a percentage share of medical bills (e.g., 20%) which an insured person must pay out-of-pocket. Deductibles are specified caps on out-of-pocket spending which an individual or family must incur before insurance begins to make payments. *See co-payments, coinsurance and deductibles.*

cost shifting – The practice of providers charging higher fees to some patients to make up for underpayment by others. The higher fees are usually charged to privately insured patients to make up for underpayment of fees for patients under Medicaid or Medicare. Cost shifting is fairly common in fee-for-service (FFS), but is extremely difficult, if not impossible, to do under managed care.

coverage – *See covered services and coverage type.*

coverage category – Classification of services, such as dental or vision, in which coverage is either fully covered, limited, restricted or not provided in a given benefit plan.

coverage effective date – The day on which a group's or subscriber's coverage begins.

coverage sequence – A benefit condition described in the benefit plan that may limit coverage on a procedure or group.

coverage type – Same as contract type. Typically, health plan subscribers can select any one of the following coverage types if listed in the schedule of eligibility. The names of the coverage type may differ from health plan to health plan, but the basic coverage type is similar:

Individual Coverage—Coverage of only an individual who has been duly accepted in the health plan. Usually, maternity care and obstetrical services are included as membership benefits, but routine newborn services are not included.

Family Coverage Type I—Coverage of the subscriber and the subscriber's spouse who have been duly accepted as members. Maternity care and obstetrical services may be included as membership benefits, as may routine newborn services.

C

Family Coverage Type II—Coverage of the subscriber and the subscriber's enrolled dependents who are his or her children, as specified. Typically, maternity care, obstetrical services and routine newborn services are membership benefits only when rendered to the subscriber, and not to the children.

Family Coverage Type III—Coverage of the subscriber, the subscriber's spouse and the subscriber's or spouse's enrolled dependents who are his or her children, as specified. Maternity care, obstetrical services and routine newborn services are usually membership benefits, but only when rendered to the subscriber or the subscriber's spouse, and not to the children.

One of the newest changes to the coverage type includes the option to include a "significant other" instead of a spouse. This option has been added to many of the health plans across the nation in response to the changing lifestyles of Americans.

covered benefit – A health care service that is considered medically necessary and is provided for under a health insurance policy. Not every medically necessary service is a covered benefit under most insurance policies. For example, custodial care may not be a covered benefit even though it may be medically necessary. *See custodial care.*

covered charge – *See covered benefit.*

covered drugs – Medications for which a health plan will reimburse a pharmacy when dispensed to a member.

covered expenses – *See covered expenses.*

covered services – Hospital, medical and miscellaneous health care expenses incurred by the insured that entitle them to a payment of benefits under a health insurance policy. Also called coverage or covered expenses.

CPHA – Commission on Professional and Hospital Activities.

CPR – *See computer-based patient record.*

CPT – *See "Current Procedural Terminology."*

CPT-4 – *Current Procedural Terminology 4th Edition. See "Current Procedural Terminology."*

CQI – *See continuous quality improvement.*

CR – *See carrier replacement.*

C

CRC – Community rating by class. *See adjusted community rating* (ACR).

credentials – Professional qualifications including professional degree, post-graduate training and education, board certification, and licensure, etc.

credentialing – The process of reviewing a practitioner's credentials for the purpose of approving his/her eligibility for hospital, PHO, or medical staff membership or participation in a health plan. Specific criteria and prerequisites are often set forth by groups such as the National Committee on Quality Assurance (NCQA) or the Joint Commission on Accreditation of Healthcare Organizations (JCAHO). The credentialing process includes a background check of a provider's training, experience or demonstrated ability, and a review of his/her records for any known disciplinary actions. Credentials and performance are periodically reviewed, which could result in a doctor's privileges being denied, modified, or withdrawn. Managed care organizations link with physicians to provide services only after an exhaustive verification of the physician's medical licenses and qualifications. Increasingly, managed care organizations are also setting standards of quality and cost-effectiveness, to which physicians must adhere.

credibility – The degree to which a group or individual account's health experience or claims expense level may be expected to repeat itself.

critical care – The specialized medical and nursing care provided to patients with life-threatening illness and single or multiple organ system failure. Care begins at the moment of illness or injury and continues throughout the patient's hospitalization and subsequent recovery. Critical care is most often provided in an intensive care unit (ICU), but can be delivered anywhere, including the scene of an accident or an operating room. *See intensive care unit.*

critical care unit – A location in the hospital where critical care (care for life-threatening illness) is provided, usually an intensive care unit (ICU). Critical care units include the medical intensive care unit (MICU), the surgical intensive care unit (SICU), the pediatric intensive care unit (PICU), the neonatal intensive care unit (NICU), coronary care unit (CCU) and the burn unit.

critical pathways – *See clinical pathways.*

CRNA – *See certified registered nurse anesthetist* (CRNA).

Current Procedural Terminology (CPT) – Currently in its 4th edition, CPT is a standardized system of terminology and coding developed

C

by the American Medical Association that is used for describing, coding and reporting medical services and procedures. The five-digit universal treatment coding system is used by physicians and other providers to identify the type and level of service provided, and is required by most insurance companies for billing purposes.

current year – The present contract year.

custodial care – Care provided primarily to assist a patient in meeting the Activities of Daily Living (ADL), not requiring skilled nursing services. Custodial care is provided primarily for the convenience of the patient or his/her family, the maintenance of the patient, or to assist the patient in meeting his or her activities of daily living, rather than primarily for therapeutic value in the treatment of a condition. Custodial care includes, but is not limited to, help in walking, bathing, dressing, eating, preparation of special diets, supervision over self-administration of medications not requiring constant attention of trained medical personnel, or acting as a companion or sitter.

Custodial care is not necessarily a membership benefit. The health plan typically has sole discretion in determining whether care is considered custodial care. As such, these health plans may consult with professional peer review committees or other appropriate sources for recommendations.

customary charge – The amount a physician normally or usually charges the majority of patients for a specific procedure.

customary, prevailing and reasonable (CPR) – A Medicare term describing a fee based on past rates and what other physicians in the area charge for similar treatment. Compare to usual, customary, and reasonable (UCR).

cycle billing – A process in which sets of accounts receivable or billing statements are produced. Each cycle pertains to a statement run. When a patient incurs new charges, the system reassigns the account to the appropriate cycle.

date of employment – The date when an employee started work. The start of coverage for health care often depends on this date.

date of service (DOS) – The date on which health care services were provided to the covered person.

day outlier – *See outlier.*

days per 1000 (DPT) – A utilization measurement of the number of days of hospital care used in a year per 1000 health plan members. This indicator is used to measure care utilization for inpatient, outpatient, residential or partial hospitalization. The basic formula is (# of days/member months) x 1000 members x # of months. Also called bed days per 1000 and visits per 1000.

DBM – Database maintenance.

DC – *See dual choice.*

DCA – *See deferred compensation administrator.*

DCI – Duplicate coverage inquiry.

DDS – *See Doctor of Dental Surgery.*

deductible – The out-of-pocket expense for covered medical services that an insured must pay before the health plan or insurance company pays benefits. Often this is a set amount for the course of a year. For example, a health plan may call for the member to pay the first $500 of covered expenses during a calendar year before reimbursement begins. Higher deductibles usually result in lower premiums.

deductible carry-over credit – Charge incurred during the last three months of a year that may be applied to the deductible and which may be carried over into the next year.

defensive medicine – Refers to the use of complete documentation primarily to guard against the risk of malpractice lawsuits.

deferred compensation administrator (DCA) – A company that provides services through retirement planning administration, third-party administration, self-insured plans, compensation planning, salary survey administration and workers compensation claims administration.

D

deferred non-emergency care – Medical or dental care (such as eye refraction, immunizations, dental prophylaxis, etc.) which can be delayed without risk to the patient.

deferred premiums – An alternative funding mechanism for companies with health plans which in effect transfers the IBNR (incurred but not reported) to the covered company's account and improves the account's cash flow by delaying the payment of monthly premiums.

Deficit Reduction Act of 1984 – States that Medicare becomes secondary for beneficiaries age 65 through 69 covered under an employer group health plan held by a working spouse who is under age 65.

DEFRA – *See Deficit Reduction Act of 1984.*

demand management – The process to match patient needs with a quality, cost-efficient setting while encouraging better member self-care.

demand-side rationing – Refers to barriers to obtaining health care by individuals who do not have sufficient income to pay for health care services or purchase health insurance.

demographic rating – A modified form of community rating which considers various characteristics such as age, sex, geographic area, and industry.

denial code – A classification system used to explain partial or total denials of claims and related services.

denial of benefits – Rejection of all or part of a claim.

dental care – Describes health care coverage for dental services and supplies, including preventive care. Dental benefits may be combined with a health insurance plan or may be a completely separate plan, possibly with another health care company.

dental care, adjunctive – Care provided to dental and oral tissue that is necessary to improve systemic (pertaining to the whole body rather than just one area) medical or surgical conditions. Adjunctive care includes oral examination and diagnosis at the request of a physician.

dental care, emergency – Care provided for the purpose of relief of oral pain, elimination of acute infection, control of life-threatening oral conditions and treatment of trauma to teeth, jaws and associated facial structures.

D

dental care, preventive – Care provided for the purpose of promoting oral health and preventing oral disease and injury.

dental clinic – A healthcare treatment facility appropriately staffed and equipped to provide outpatient dental care that may include a wide range of specialized and consultative support.

dental service – Provision of services providing preventive care, diagnosis, and treatment of patients to promote, maintain or restore dental health.

dental treatment facility (DTF) – *See dental clinic.*

dental treatment room (DTR) – A properly outfitted room including a dental chair, dental unit and dental light where clinical dental procedures are performed.

dentist – Person qualified by a degree in dental surgery (DDS) or dental medicine (DMD). *See Doctor of Dental Surgery or Doctor of Dental Medicine.*

department number – A number used to indicate business segments within an employer company. Typically used when billing is generated through each business segment.

department of insurance (DOI) – The branch of state government charged with regulating the insurance industry, issuing insurance licenses, conducting market surveillance, etc.

dependent – A subscriber's spouse and dependent children under the limiting age of the contract. In some health plans, dependents may include those unmarried dependents who become disabled prior to the limiting age.

dependent age limitation – The age at which coverage ceases for a dependent child covered under a family membership.

dermatology – The diagnosis and treatment of skin diseases and disorders.

designated health services (DHS) – Eleven types of healthcare services that the Stark II laws prohibit from referral by a physician who has a financial relationship with another health care entity (e.g., facility, provider, etc.). *See Stark and Stark II Laws.* The DHS's covered by the law are:

1. clinical laboratory
2. physical therapy (including speech-language pathology services)
3. occupational therapy

D

4. radiology, (including magnetic resonance imaging, computerized axial tomography scans and ultrasound)
5. radiation therapy services and supplies
6. durable medical equipment and supplies
7. parenteral and enteral nutrients, equipment, and supplies
8. prosthetics, orthotics, and prosthetic devices and supplies
9. home health services
10. outpatient prescription drugs
11. inpatient and outpatient hospital services.

designated hospital – A hospital under contract with a health plan to provide services to the plan's members. Members generally save money by using a designated hospital for emergency services rather than a non-designated hospital. *See in-network and out-of-network.*

designated mental health provider – Person or place authorized by a health plan to provide or suggest appropriate mental health and substance abuse care.

developmental disability – Mental retardation or a related condition. A severe, chronic disability manifested during the developmental period which results in impaired intellectual functioning or deficiencies in essential skills. *See also mental retardation, related condition.*

DHS – *See designated health services.*

diagnosis – The identification of a condition or disease and the nature of its cause. Diagnosis includes distinguishing one disease from another, the concise technical description of the condition and its cause, and the appropriate code (ICD-9-CM and DRG).

Diagnosis and Statistical Manual (DSMIII-R) – The American Psychiatric Association's manual of diagnostic criteria and terminology, widely accepted as the common language of mental health clinicians and researchers. The 3rd Edition—Revised is currently in use.

diagnosis code – *See diagnostic code.*

diagnosis-related groups (DRGs) – A system of classification for inpatient hospital services based on principal diagnosis, secondary diagnosis, surgical procedures, age, sex and presence of complications. This system of classification clusters patients into 468 categories and is used as a financing mechanism to reimburse hospitals and selected providers for services rendered. As such, it is one form of a case rate payment system.

The DRG classification system was developed at Yale University

D

using 383 major diagnostic categories based on the ICD-9 codes, and was instituted by Medicare for the payment of hospital services. All Medicare inpatient hospital operating costs are determined in advance and paid on a per-case basis, according to fixed amount or weight established for each DRG. DRGs were originally designed to facilitate the utilization review process, but are also used to analyze patient case mix in hospitals and determine hospital and other providers' reimbursement policy. Also called diagnostic related groups.

diagnostic admission – Refers to an inpatient hospital admission that is primarily for diagnostic purposes.

diagnostic code – A numerical identification as listed in the ICD (*International Classification of Diseases*) of a condition, cause or disease.

diagnostic services – X-ray, laboratory, and pathology services that are specifically used to diagnose a condition, illness or injury.

direct contracting – Individual employers or business coalitions contract directly with providers for health care services, eliminating the need for a managed care company or insurance intermediary. Direct contracting enables employers to include in the plan the specific services preferred by their employees (usually done under ERISA guidelines). Since providers are usually at full risk in a direct contracting situation, the key is to price services correctly. Ideally, direct contracting is best done by a very strong integrated delivery system (IDS) or accountable health plan (AHP). *See Employee Retirement Income Security Act (ERISA), integrated delivery system and accountable health plan.*

direct pay – A method of billing subscribers directly for the premium payments of their health plan. Members are billed and pay dues direct to their health care plans. Direct pay rates are usually higher than group rates. Direct pay members typically consist of group conversion, nongroup, sponsored and a few group-affiliated members as a special accommodation. Also called billed direct or billed-at-home.

direct payment subscriber – A person enrolled in a health plan who pays premiums directly to the plan rather than through a group. Rates of payment are generally higher, and benefits may not be as extensive as for the subscriber enrolled and paying as a member of the group.

D

disability – Any limitation of physical, mental or social activity as compared with other individuals of similar age, sex, and occupation. *See total disability, long-term disability insurance, and short-term disability.*

disability insurance – Reimbursement that pays weekly or monthly for lost income due to a temporary or permanent illness or injury (disability). Sometimes called disability income insurance.

disallowance – The amount of a provider's fee that is above a payer's (e.g., health plan's) fee ceiling or maximum allowable, and which the payer will not recognize for payment.

discharge – Formal release by a hospital of a patient who no longer requires inpatient care, or of a patient who voluntarily departs the hospital. The day of discharge is the day the hospital formally terminates hospitalization.

discharge diagnosis – Any one of the diagnoses recorded and studied after all data are collected in the course of a patient's stay.

discharge planning – A program to facilitate early, safe release from the hospital by planning and providing the patient's needed medical services after discharge from the inpatient facility. Required by Medicare and JCAHO for all hospital patients.

discharge summary – A report prepared by a physician or clinician at the end of a patient's hospital stay summarizing the diagnosis, treatment and results, and outlining any recommendations following discharge. *See discharge planning.*

discount – As established in a provider contract, the discount is the percentage deducted during adjudication from the allowed amount on a claim to be paid to a provider.

discounted fee-for-service (discounted FFS) – A way of paying providers using negotiated discounts. In discounted FFS, the physician's services are still provided as fee-for-service (FFS), but at a negotiated rate less than their usual fee. This may be a fixed amount per service or a percentage discount. Providers generally accept such contracts because they represent a means to increase their volume or reduce their chances of losing volume.

discrepancy notice – A formal notification between a health plan and a provider (physician or hospital) indicating an inconsistency between their records regarding the disposition of a patient. The discrepancy can be anything from the group number to differences in claim amounts.

D

disease management – Programs that follow specific diseases/conditions and their treatments, as well as introduce treatment protocols in an effort to optimize beneficial outcomes that reduce the cost of care. Most often associated with large pharmaceutical companies, in conjunction with physicians, that maintain databases of prescribed medications used in treating these diseases and conditions. Disease management programs exist for such maladies as asthma, diabetes, depression and lipid disorders.

Disease management identifies patient populations with acute and chronic diseases and introduces interventions throughout the lifecycle of the disease that focuses on prevention of recurrence, improved quality of life and cost-effective care. The outcomes of the interventions are scrutinized via measurement and research to ensure the approach is making a positive impact. Sometimes called population-based care management or care mapping. *See disease state management, outcomes management and outcomes research.*

disease prevention – *See preventive care.*

disease state management – The management of a patient's entire disease state, rather than treating individual components of a disease in isolation. Emphasis is placed on beneficial outcomes and cost-effectiveness. Disease state management considers how best to treat the patient's overall condition, taking into account all foreseeable side effects and treatment costs.

disenrollment – Refers to the occurrence of individuals or groups leaving a health care plan or changing health care providers.

dispensing fee – A fee charged for filling a prescription, frequently used in pharmacy, vision, and hearing programs.

disproportionate share (DISPRO or DSH) – A program which provides additional reimbursement to hospitals which serve a disproportionate share of low-income patients to compensate for revenues lost by serving needy populations. A disproportionate share facility receives additional Medicaid funds in consideration of providing a high volume of care to low-income persons.

disproportionate share hospital – A hospital which serves a higher than average number of Medicaid and other low-income patients. The facility receives additional Medicaid funds in consideration of providing a high volume of care to low-income persons.

distribution channels – Refers to the way health plans and services are delivered. The distribution channels would include, for example,

D

brokers and agents for insurance, pharmacies and pharmaceutical companies for drugs, and physicians and other clinicians for health care.

DMD – *See Doctor of Dental Medicine.*

DME – *See durable medical equipment.*

DN – *See discrepancy notice.*

DOB – Date of birth.

Doctor of Chiropractic (DC) – *See chiropractor.*

Doctor of Dental Surgery (DDS) – Commonly called a dentist, a person duly trained and educated in a dental program and licensed by the state to practice the prevention and treatment of diseases of the teeth and mouth.

Doctor of Dental Medicine (DMD) – Commonly called a dentist, a person duly trained and educated in a dental program and licensed by the state to practice the prevention and treatment of diseases of the teeth and mouth.

Doctor of Medicine (MD) – A person duly trained and educated at a conventional medical school and licensed by the state to practice medicine.

Doctor of Optometry (OD) – Often referred to as an optometrist, a person duly trained and educated in the testing and correction of vision problems at an optometric school and licensed by the state.

Doctor of Osteopathy (DO) – Often referred to as an osteopath, a person duly trained and educated in the diagnosis and treatment of bone diseases at an osteopathic medical school and licensed by the state. The length and intensity of education and training for osteopaths is similar to that of conventional medical schools, and in many states they are licensed as M.D.s as well as Osteopaths. Osteopathic education was originally based on manipulation of the human structure, but evolved into the same training and background as conventional medical schools with similar requirements.

Doctor of Podiatric Medicine (DPM) – Often referred to as a podiatrist, a person duly trained and educated at a school of podiatry in the diagnosis and treatment of diseases and disorders of the feet. Podiatrists are licensed by the state. Podiatrists are sometimes called chiropodists, although this is now considered an obsolete term.

D

doctor's office care – Care rendered in a doctor's office which usually does not include surgery.

DOH – Department of Health.

DOI – Department of Insurance.

domiciliary care – *See adult foster care and assisted living center.*

donor – A person who gives, donates, or contributes; for example, an organ or blood donor.

DOS – Date of Service.

downcoding – Occurs when a provider (hospital, physician, etc.) submits a bill to a payer (e.g., insurance company, managed care organization, etc.) with an invalid procedure code. The payer identifies that the code is no longer valid and, using the physical description of the procedure performed, selects the procedure code that pays the least for that description. Consequently, downcoding can cost a provider lost revenue.

downtime – The period during which a computer, communications line, or other device is malfunctioning because of mechanical or electronic failure.

DPM – *See Doctor of Podiatric Medicine.*

DPT – *See days per 1000 (thousand).*

DPR – *See drug price review.*

DRG – *See diagnosis related groups.*

DRG weight – An index number which reflects the relative resource consumption associated with each DRG.

drug formulary – In its most basic definition, a listing of medications covered by a benefit plan and dispensed through participating pharmacies. The listing is usually developed by a health plan's pharmacy and therapeutics (P&T) committee. Formularies may be "open or voluntary," in which case the drugs on it are preferred but not required; or "closed, select or mandatory," in which only formulary drugs are covered. Sometimes, non-formulary drugs can be covered if proper authorization is obtained beforehand and there is a strong medical reason. The formulary is subject to periodic review and modification by the health plan. *See open formulary, closed formulary and restricted formulary.*

D

drug price review (DPR) – A weekly updating of drug prices, at average wholesale price (AWP), from the *American Druggist Blue Book*. *See maximum allowable cost list.*

drug provider – A pharmacy, physician or other licensed health care professional licensed to dispense prescription drugs.

drug use evaluation (DUE) – Same as drug utilization review, only qualitative in nature. *See drug utilization review.*

drug utilization review (DUR) – A review of prescription drug use and physician prescribing patterns to determine the appropriateness of drug treatment. DUR can be for an individual patient or for an entire insured population, and may be performed on a concurrent (current usage), retrospective (past usage) or prospective (future usage) basis.

In a review for an individual patient, the primary goal is to make sure that the patient's medications are not adversely interacting with one another, and to consider other factors that may affect drug usage, like allergies. In reviewing an entire population, the goal may be to find ways to reduce costs while maintaining effective drug therapy. Cost reduction methods may include substituting generic drugs for name brands and using a drug formulary.

DSH – *See disproportionate share hospital.*

DSM – *See disease-state management.*

DSMIII-R – *See diagnosis and statistical manual.*

DTF – Dental treatment facility.

DTR – Dental treatment room.

dual choice (DC) – An arrangement where an employer offers a choice of two or more types of health coverage to employees. For example, an HMO and PPO, or an HMO and an indemnity plan. Section 1310 of the HMO Act provides for dual choice. Also called multiple choice or dual option.

dual eligibles – Individuals who are eligible for both Medicare and Medicaid.

DUE – *See drug-use evaluation.*

due date – The date when payment should be received in the health plan's office.

dues – Payments required in order to maintain membership.

D

dummy application – When a health plan is enrolling a new company, there are times when an employee cannot be contacted by the employer to complete the membership application. In such cases, the company may complete the application for the employee and submit it unsigned. The group processing department of the health plan will include this temporary dummy application to verify group eligibility, determine the required enrollment percentage, and verify rates based on final enrollment. Any adjustments to the application can be made when the employee returns to work.

duplication of benefits – Occurs when a person is covered under more than one health insurance policy and may collect payments for the same hospital or medical expenses from more than one insurer. Also known as multiple coverage.

Some health policies have anti-duplication clauses, but most states will not allow group health policies to apply these clauses to individual insurance. Where duplication exists with a group anti-duplication clause, the group insurer responsible for paying its benefits first is considered the primary payer.

duplicate coverage inquiry (DCI) – A request to a health insurance or managed care company by another health insurance or managed care company to find out whether other coverage exists for the purpose of coordination of benefits. *See coordination of benefits.*

DUR – *See drug utilization review.*

durable medical equipment (DME) – Equipment that meets the following criteria:

- is primarily and customarily used to serve a medical purpose;
- generally, is not useful in the absence of illness or injury;
- can withstand repeated use;
- is appropriate for use in the home.

Examples of durable medical equipment include hospital beds, wheelchairs, crutches and oxygen equipment.

DX – Abbreviation for diagnosis code.

E & M codes – CPT-4 codes that describe patient encounters with health care professionals for the purpose of Evaluation and Management of general health status. *See "Current Procedural Terminology"* (CPT).

EAP – *See employee assistance program.*

early and periodic screening, diagnosis, and treatment (EPSDT) – The EPSDT program covers screening and diagnostic services to determine physical or mental defects in recipients under age 21, as well as health care and other measures to correct or ameliorate any defects and chronic conditions discovered.

earned income – *See earned premiums.*

earned premiums – Premiums or benefits paid which have been allocated to the proper earned period.

EBT/EFT – Electronic benefit transfer / electronic funds transfer. An automated alternative to paper checks which involves direct payment from one account to another. For example, from a patient's checking account directly to the accounts receivable of the doctor's office.

ECF – *See extended care facility.*

E codes – ICD-9 codes for external causes of injury and poisoning that explain how the injury occurred.

economic credentialing – Describes taking a physician's economic behavior into account (i.e., tests ordered, hospital bed days, outcomes, etc.) as part of the credentialing process. *See credentialing.*

EDI – *See electronic data interchange.*

EDP – Electronic data processing.

effective date (insurance) – The date on which the membership, coverage or rate become becomes effective.

efficacy – The effectiveness of a medical procedure or intervention. If a treatment or service produces a health benefit, it is considered efficacious or effective.

elective abortion – Any nonspontaneous abortion (termination of pregnancy) for any reason other than to prevent the death of the female upon whom the abortion is performed.

E

elective care – Medical, surgical, or dental care which, in the opinion of professional authority, could be performed at another time or place without jeopardizing the patient's life, limb, health or well-being. Examples include surgery for cosmetic purposes, vitamins without a therapeutic basis, sterilization procedures, elective abortions, procedures for dental prosthesis and prosthetic appliances.

elective surgery – Surgery which needs not be performed on an emergency basis because reasonable delays will not affect the outcome of surgery unfavorably. Elective surgery is usually necessary and may be major.

electronic claim – A digital representation of a medical bill generated by a provider or by the provider's billing agent for submission to a health insurance payer using telecommunications.

electronic data interchange (EDI) – The electronic exchange of claims, referrals, pre-certifications, utilization data and other health care related information utilizing computers.

electronic fund transfers (EFT) – The transfer of money between businesses and individuals by use of computer-generated debit and credit entries rather than checks or cash. Progressive health care companies are either using or developing EFTs for Medicaid and Medicare billing.

electronic medical record (EMR) – Describes the technology where medical records are kept on computer rather than in paper files. EMR would supply providers with real-time clinical data storage and access. When fully developed, EMR could allow health care entities to share data for medical outcome studies, speed up claims processing, and improve the quality and efficiency of care.

eligibility date – The date an individual and/or dependents become eligible for benefits under an employee benefit plan.

eligibility for coverage (in group membership) – The criteria that a person must meet to gain coverage through a group such as age, employment status, continued employment, etc.

eligibility guarantee – An assurance of reimbursement to the medical group for services/goods provided to a member who subsequently is found to be ineligible for benefits.

eligibility verification – The process a health plan goes through to confirm that the claimant is an active member of the plan prior to authorizing payment for services.

E

eligibility waiting period – The length of time the employee must be employed by his/her employer before being eligible for coverage. Also referred to as probationary period.

eligible dependents – Persons entitled to apply for and maintain membership in a health plan under a member's family coverage.

eligible employee – An employee who qualifies to receive health plan benefits.

eligible expenses – Charges that are covered under a health plan. *See also covered services and approved services.*

eligible person – A person entitled to apply for and maintain membership in a health plan as specified in the plan contract.

elimination period – *See waiting period.*

emergency – A severe or life-threatening condition that requires immediate medical intervention (within minutes or hours), and if not treated immediately, would threaten or impair the health of a patient. In an HMO, an emergency may be the only acceptable reason for hospital admission without precertification.

emergency center – Non-hospital-affiliated health facility that provides short-term care for minor medical emergencies or procedures needing immediate treatment. Also called urgent center (urgi-center), or free-standing emergency medical service center.

emergency department (ED) – *See emergency room (ER).*

emergency medicine – The branch of medicine dealing with medical and surgical emergencies, usually in a hospital emergency room (department).

emergency room (ER) – An area of a hospital specifically designed to treat patients that require immediate medical attention for a trauma or unforeseen acute illness. The ER is where most of the abuse in health care occurs, as people often use the ER for simple problems and procedures that could have easily been done in a primary care physician's (PCP) office. For example, non-life threatening cuts, broken bones or high fevers. In defense of this behavior, it should be noted that ERs are sometimes the only place to get health care services 24 hours a day and after typical physician office hours. Also called emergency department (ED).

emergency services – Services provided in connection with an unforeseen acute illness or injury requiring immediate medical attention. Emergency services are provided 24 hours a day. The JCAHO

E

accreditation manual classifies emergency services at three levels as follows:

Level I Emergency Service—Requires at least one physician experienced in emergency care on duty in the emergency care area. There must be in-hospital physician coverage by members of the medical staff or by senior-level residents for at least medical, surgical, orthopedic, obstetrical, gynecological, pediatric and anesthesiology services. When such coverage can be demonstrated to be met suitably through another mechanism, an equivalency will be considered to exist for purposes of compliance with the requirement. Other specialty consultation must be available within approximately 30 minutes. Initial consultation through two-way voice communication is acceptable. The hospital's scope of services must include inhouse capabilities for managing physical and related emotional problems on a definitive basis.

Level II Emergency Service—Requires at least one physician experienced in emergency care on duty in the emergency care area. Specialty consultation must be available within approximately 30 minutes by members of the medical staff or by senior-level residents. Initial consultation through two-way voice communication is acceptable. The hospital's scope of services must include inhouse capabilities for managing physical and related emotional problems, with provision for patient transfer to another facility when needed.

Level III Emergency Service—Requires at least one physician available to the emergency care area from within the hospital who is available immediately through two-way voice communication. Specialty consultation must be available by request of the attending medical staff member or by transfer to a designated hospital where definitive care can be provided.

emergent conditions – Refers to any physical condition that requires immediate medical attention, is potentially threatening to life or function, and is harmful if treatment is delayed.

emergi-center – *See emergency center.*

emerging healthcare organizations (EHO) – Refers to hospitals and physicians (and sometimes payers) that are in the process of integrating or merging to meet the market's health care needs and remain economically viable.

employee assistance program (EAP) – A term used for employer-sponsored counseling services designed to assist employees and

E

their families in finding solutions for workplace and personal problems. The intent of such programs is to reduce the rate of absenteeism and employee turnover and increase productivity by eliminating issues that affect a company's performance.

Depending on the employer, EAP services may include assistance for legal or financial problems, childcare, eldercare, substance abuse, stress issues and sexual harassment. EAP programs can also provide referrals for employees who may need treatment. Most EAPs are run by either a managed care organization or as a carve-out by a managed behavioral health company.

employee benefit plan – Any indirect form of compensation. Under ERISA (Employee Retirement Income Security Act), an employee benefit plan is defined as any form of pension plan or welfare plan.

Employee Retirement Income Security Act of 1974, Public Law 93-406 (ERISA) – A federal government act that protects employee pensions and fringe benefits. The law mandates reporting and disclosure requirements for group life and health plans, and establishes rules regarding group program of benefits for employees including: participation, crediting of service, vesting, communication and disclosure, funding and fiduciary conduct.

ERISA exempts self-insured health plans from state laws governing health insurance, including contribution to risk pools, prohibitions against disease discrimination, and other state health reforms. Also called the Pension Reform Act.

employer mandate – Refers to some state laws that require employers to pay a share of their employees' health coverage.

Until 1995, employer mandate described a condition when, under the Federal HMO Act, federally qualified HMOs could require an employer to offer at least one HMO plan to their employees.

employer self-insured programs – See *self-insurance or self-insured.*

enabling services – Services that ease patient access to health care, such as transportation or translation services.

encounter – A face-to-face member visit to a provider. If more than one evaluation or treatment takes place during the same visit, it is still considered one encounter. For instance, there may be a variety of services performed at an encounter, including a brief office visit, an EKG, a lab test and an immunization.

encounter fee – A fee which is charged to a health plan participant by

E

a preferred provider each time care is rendered in either a preferred provider hospital emergency room or in the office of the preferred provider. The amount of the fee is generally set forth in the schedule of benefits.

encounter form – Form generated when a patient receives services containing patient demographics, services rendered (CPT) and diagnosis (ICD) codes.

endocrinology – Branch of internal medicine dealing with diseases of the ductless glands (thyroid, parathyroid, pituitary, adrenals, pancreas, ovaries, and testes).

endorsement –
1. A contractual statement, imprinted upon a certificate, that validates and/or defines a certificate.
2. A provision added to a contract or certificate issued by the insurer which changes the terms therein.

enrolled dependents – Those eligible dependents who have applied for enrollment under a member's family coverage and who have been accepted for such enrollment by the health care plan.

enrolled group – Persons with the same employer or with membership in an organization in common, who are enrolled collectively in a health plan. Also called contract group.

enrollee – Any person eligible as either a subscriber or a dependent covered under a health care plan. Also known as beneficiary or member, including those who have enrolled (subscribed) and their eligible dependents.

enrollment –
1. The process by which a health plan signs up individuals or groups as subscribers, including the entry of an individual's membership information in the health plan's computer system. Essentially, individuals are "enrolled" as members into prepaid plans.
2. The number of members in a health plan, or the number of members assigned to a physician or medical group providing care under contract with a health plan.

enrollment area – The geographic area within which subscribers must live to be enrolled in the health plan.

enrollment card – A document signed by an employee stating his/her interest in participating in the benefits of a group insurance plan.

E

enrollment date – The date coverage begins for a participant as assigned by the managed care company.

enrollment period – Period during which individuals may enroll for life insurance or health coverage benefits. Most contributory group insurance has an annual enrollment period when members of the group may elect to begin contributing and become covered.

enrollment regulations – A health plan's rules for determining eligibility for enrollment.

ENT – An abbreviation for ear, nose and throat. *See otolaryngologist.*

environmental services – Services such as housekeeping, laundry, maintenance and liquid and solid waste control performed to ensure safe, sanitary and efficient hospital operation.

EOB – *See explanation of benefits.*

EOI – *See evidence of insurability.*

EOM – End of month.

EOMB – *See explanation of Medicare benefits.*

EOY – End of year.

episode of care – A term used to describe and measure the various health care services and encounters received by a patient in connection with a particular medical problem or situation. Also called an episode of hospital care.

EPMPY – Encounters per member per year.

EPO – *See exclusive provider organization.*

EPSDT – *See Early and Periodic Screening, Diagnosis and Treatment.*

ERISA – *See Employee Retirement Income Security Act of 1974.*

evaluation and management services (E/M) – Patient evaluation and management functions performed during patient office visits, outpatient visits and hospital visits or consultations. They consist of taking a patient history, performing a patient examination and the cognitive medical decision-making.

evergreen contracts – Managed care contracts that automatically renew themselves after the initial term (usually one year) has been completed.

evidence-based medicine (EBM) – The practice of integrating both clinical expertise and the best available external evidence to make

E

decisions about the care of individual patients. In EBM, physicians formulate a clinical question, research the answer to the question, combine the results from the research with their clinical expertise and apply this knowledge to treating the patient.

evidence of coverage (EOC) – *See explanation of coverage* (EOC).

evidence of insurability (EOI) – Any statement or proof of a person's physical condition or occupation that affects his/her eligibility for insurance coverage. The proof is usually a written statement such as an application form, and is required for eligibles who do not enroll during an open enrollment period. Also called evidence of good health.

exceptions – *See exclusions.*

excess insurance – Insurance that pays over and above the primary amount of coverage.

excess risk – Either specific or aggregate stop-loss coverage.

exclusions – Specific conditions or services listed in the employee benefit plan that are not covered by the terms of the health plan. Also called exceptions.

exclusive provider organization (EPO) – An EPO is similar to a PPO in that physicians do not receive capitated payments, but it provides benefit coverage only through contracted providers. If patients elect to seek care outside of the network, then they will usually not be reimbursed for the cost of the treatment. This is why it is called "exclusive." The EPO is also similar to an HMO because it has a limited provider network and makes use of a utilization management system.

exclusivity clause – A part of a contract which prohibits physicians from contracting with more than one managed care organization (e.g., HMO, PPO, or POS).

expansion – Refers to the growth of a health plan's network either geographically or in the number of hospitals and providers it will add.

expected incurred claims – The dollar amount of claims attributable to a particular period of time that are expected to be paid.

experience – The extent of usage of health plan benefits by members. Describes the relationship of premium to claims for health plan benefits for a stated time period. Usually expressed as a percent or ratio.

E

experience period – A period of time (normally 12 months) during which premium and claim records are accumulated for the purpose of a rate review.

experience-rated premium – A premium based upon the experience rating and subject to periodic adjustment in line with actual claims or utilization experience.

experience rating – A method of evaluating the risk of an individual or group by looking at the applicant's health history. Age, sex, and health care utilization experience are the principal determinants in rate setting using this method. Typically, companies with sicker workers pay higher premiums. Experience rating is not allowed for federally-qualified HMOs. Compare to community rating.

experimental or investigative care – Care which has not been generally accepted as standard care according to the prevalent standards of medical care practice, or any care requiring federal or other governmental agency approval not granted at the time the care was rendered.

explanation of benefits (EOB) – A statement issued to a member by their health plan listing services provided, amount billed, dollars covered by benefits, and payment made.

explanation of coverage (EOC) – A booklet provided by the carrier to the insured summarizing benefits under an insurance plan.

explanation of review (EOR) – A statement issued to providers by their health plan listing services rendered, amount billed, amount paid and any disallowances.

explanation of Medicare benefits (EOMB) – A form issued to persons eligible for Medicare Part B benefit consideration by the Medicare carrier. If the physician has not accepted an assignment with Medicare and benefits are available, the Medicare benefit check payable to the patient will accompany the form.

exposure –
1. The state of being subject to a chance of loss.
2. The number of contracts exposed to the chance of loss for the duration of a specific period.

extended benefits –
1. Benefits provided in excess of basic health care plans.
2. Extension of benefits for limited periods after termination of plan coverage.

E

extended care facility (ECF) – A specifically qualified facility which is staffed and equipped to furnish skilled nursing care as well as rehabilitation and convalescent services to patients whose conditions do not require general hospital care. Such facilities must be licensed as such by the state where they operate. *See skilled nursing facility* (SNF).

extension of benefits – Insurance policy provision that allows medical coverage to continue past termination of employment. *See also* COBRA.

external quality review organization (EQRO) – A quality assurance entity that performs an annual review of the quality of services furnished by each Health Maintenance Organization (HMO) or health insuring organization (HIO) that contracts with a state. The EQRO must be independent of the state where it is conducting reviews.

E-Z claim – A three-part claim form which serves both as a charge/receipt form and an instant insurance claim. Compare to superbill.

FA – *See fiscal agent - Medicaid.*

facility – User-defined building area from which a provider may render services.

facility specific – Rate methodology which pays providers delivering the same type of service at different rates. Rates are tied explicitly to facility expenditures on items most directly related to patient care.

faculty practice plan – A form of group practice where the faculty of a medical school provide patient care in addition to their teaching and research responsibilities.

family deductible – The initial amount that must be paid by the covered member family before insurance benefits will be reimbursed. The family deductible is usually equal to two or three times the individual deductible, and once the family deductible for a calendar year is satisfied, no further individual deductibles must be satisfied in that calendar year.

Family Medical Leave Act (FMLA) – Passed in 1993, the Act requires employers with 50 or more employees to provide an employee 12 weeks of leave per year for birth or adoption of a child, or to care for a sick family member. FMLA also requires the employers to provide 12 weeks of leave for an employee with a serious health condition, defined as an "illness, injury, or impairment of physical or mental condition." The condition must involve either continuing treatment by a provider or inpatient care.

family membership – A health plan covering a subscriber and one or more dependents.

family practitioner – Physicians who provide medical care to all age groups. Family practitioners' services often include internal medicine, pediatrics, and some surgery.

favorable selection – Selection of subscribers or covered lives based on data which shows a tendency for utilization of health services in that population group to be lower than expected or estimated. *See cherry picking.*

federal employee program (FEP) – The government-wide service benefits program for employees of the federal government.

F

federal qualification – Federal designation that allows an organization to participate in certain Medicare cost and risk contracts. The federally qualified designation also allows those organizations to receive federal grants and loans. *See federally qualified health center and federally qualified HMO.*

federally qualified health center (FQHC) – A health center eligible for a cost-based reimbursement rate from Medicare and Medicaid. The FQHC designation is usually given to qualified providers in medically underserved areas, and allows for the direct reimbursement of nurse practitioners, physician assistants and certified nurse midwives. Most FQHCs are located in the inner cities or rural areas and include community health centers, migrant health centers, and health care for the homeless. FQHC services may include comprehensive primary and preventive services, health education and mental health services.

federally qualified HMO – An HMO that meets certain federally stipulated provisions aimed at protecting consumer (e.g., providing a broad range of basic health services, assuring financial solvency, and monitoring the quality of care). HMOs must apply to the federal government for qualification, where the process is administered by the Health Care Financing Administration (HCFA) under the Department of Health and Human Services (HHS).

The Health Maintenance Organization Act of 1973 encouraged the development of HMOs. Under this act, HMOs that voluntarily chose to comply with regulatory requirements more stringent than state law (federally-qualified HMOs) are eligible to receive federal grants, loans and loan guarantees not available to non-qualified plans. Until recently, employers of 25 or more workers were required to offer a federally-qualified HMO if the plan requested to be included in the company's health benefits program.

federal Medicaid managed care waiver program – The process used by states to receive permission to implement managed care programs for their Medicaid or other categorically eligible beneficiaries. *See Section 1115 Medicaid Waiver.*

federal medical assistance percentage (FMAP) – The percentage of federal dollars available to a state to provide Medicaid services. FMAP is calculated annually based on a formula designed to provide a higher federal matching rate to states with lower per capita income. In 1994 the FMAP for Texas was approximately 64 percent for most services. The federal share of Medicaid administrative costs is not based on a per capita income formula. It is a flat 50

F

percent for most activities.

fee – A charge or price for professional services.

fee disclosure – Refers to physicians and other health care providers discussing their fees with patients prior to treatment.

fee-for-service (FFS) – The traditional method for financing health services where physicians and hospitals are paid for each service they provide. No prepayment is involved; however, discounts have been established in managed care plans (discounted fee-for-service). Fee-for-service is the system used by indemnity health plans (where individuals pay 100% of all medical bills up to an annual deductible). This traditional method contrasts with that used in the prepaid sector where services are covered by a fixed payment made in advance that is independent of the number of services rendered. Also known as fee-for-service reimbursement.

fee-for-service equivalency – A quantitative measure of the difference between the amount a physician or other health care provider receives from an alternative reimbursement system, such as capitation, compared to fee-for-service reimbursement.

fee-for-service reimbursement – See *fee-for-service*.

fee schedule – A listing of fees or allowances for specified medical or health procedures, which usually represents the maximum amounts the health plan will pay for specified procedures. Fee schedule rates are usually considerably less than billed charges. Sometimes called a table of allowances.

FEHBP – Federal Employee Health Benefits Program.

FEHBP members – Federal Employee Health Benefits Program members.

FFP – Federal financial participation.

FFS – See *fee-for-service*.

FICA – Federal Insurance Contribution Act.

fiduciary – One, who without regard for personal interests, has an obligation to act on behalf of another individual. For example, a physician has a fiduciary relationship with patients. With the entry of managed care into health care, that fiduciary relationship may be in jeopardy. Under certain circumstances, providers may have to perform procedures, treatments or tests that are not always covered under the patient's plan. Those services are paid out of the

F

provider's pocket, and could make it more difficult to act on the patient's best interest.

FIFO – First in first out. A queuing technique in which the next item to be retrieved is the oldest item (or first item) in the queue.

FIG – Fiscal intermediary group.

first-dollar coverage – Coverage usually under a health or casualty insurance program which begins paying with the first dollar of expense incurred by the insured for the covered benefits. Such coverage, therefore, has no deductibles although it may have copayments or coinsurance.

first pass – A claim that has adjudicated (the process to decide whether to pay or reject) completely from data entry to payment or denial without getting suspended (stopped for any reason). *See adjudication*. Also called pass through.

fiscal agent - Medicaid – Fiscal agent - Medicaid's fiscal intermediary; operates the provider claims system and MMIS database.

fiscal intermediary – In general, the company that has contracted with providers to process claims for reimbursement under health care coverage. However, the term is usually applied to contractors performing claim processing, communications, audits and other administrative duties for Medicare, particularly under Part A.

fiscal soundness – The requirement that managed care organizations have sufficient operating funds on hand, or available in reserve, to cover all expenses associated with services for which they have assumed financial risk.

fiscal year – Any 12-month period for which annual accounts are kept. Sometimes, but by no means necessarily, the same as a calendar year. Any 12-month period used by government or a business entity for its annual financial accounting cycle.

fixed costs – Costs which do not change with fluctuations in census or in utilization of services.

flat fee-per-case – A flat fee paid to a provider to cover all services for a patient's treatment based on diagnosis (episode of care). Flat fee-per-case is sometimes a precursor to capitation. Under flat fee-per-case, providers accept considerable risk, but have flexibility in how to meet patients' needs. To reduce their risk, providers have to negotiate favorable case rates with insurance companies and acquire enough patients to make the risk acceptable. Also called

F

bundled rate or case rate.

flat rate – Reimbursement methodology in which all providers delivering the same service are paid at the same rate. Also known as uniform rate.

flexible benefit plan – Program offered by some employers in which employees may choose among a number of health care benefit options. *See also cafeteria plan.*

flexible spending account (FSA) – A plan which provides employees a choice between taxable cash and non-taxable benefits for unreimbursed health care expenses or dependent care expenses. This plan qualifies under Section 125 of the IRS Code. *See also medical spending account.*

formatting and protocol standards – Data exchange standards which are needed between CPR systems (computer-based patient record), as well as the CPR and other provider systems, to ensure uniformity in how data is collected, stored and presented.   Proactive providers are current in their knowledge of these standards and are working to make sure that their data systems conform to these standards. *See computer-based patient record* (CPR).

formulary – *See drug formulary.*

foundation – *See medical foundation.*

FQHC – *See federally qualified health center (or clinic).*

fraud – Intentional misrepresentation by either providers or consumers to obtain services, obtain payment for services, or claim program eligibility.

freedom of choice – In Medicaid, it is when a state must ensure that Medicaid beneficiaries are free to obtain services from any qualified provider. Exceptions are possible through waivers of Medicaid and special contract options.

In commercial health insurance, freedom of choice refers to the ability of members to go to whomever they want for health care, especially without the need for a referral. Indemnity plans offer the most freedom of choice; closed access HMOs offer the least.

free-standing surgical center – A health care facility staffed by licensed physicians designed to handle surgical procedures that do not require overnight hospital care.

FSA – Flexible spending account.

F

full disability – A classification of disability under which the patient has lost full capacity to earn a living.

full-risk capitation – Describes a reimbursement method where a health plan provides all health care services to an enrolled population including hospitalization, preventive care, home care, dental care, mental health services, etc. By doing so, the health plan accepts all risk for that population, meaning that they need to keep costs for providing health care below the amount of premiums they take in. *See capitation, risk and premium.*

full-time equivalent (FTE) – Work force equivalent of one individual working full-time for a specific period, which may be made up of several part-time individuals or one full-time individual.

fully insured – A health care funding mechanism where the insurer assumes all risk (responsibility for the reimbursement of medical expenses incurred by group members) and the insured group assumes none. Premiums are typically slightly higher than if the group assumes some or all of the risk.

functional costs – Operating costs classified by function. The two primary functions being claims administration expenses (CAE) and general office expenses (GOE).

funding level – Amount of revenue required to finance a medical care program.

funding method – A system for employers to pay for health benefit plans. The most common methods include prospective and/or retrospective premium payment, shared risk arrangement and self-funding. *See also self-insured, risk and premium.*

gag clause – A provision of a contract between a managed care organization and a health care provider that restricts the amount of information a provider may share with a patient, or that limits the circumstances under which a provider may recommend a specific treatment option.

gain from operations – Surplus of total income over benefit and administrative expenses.

gaming – Refers to an attempt to manipulate "the system" in an illegal or unethical manner. The terms "gaming" and "to game the system" are used, for example, in connection with efforts to bill under the prospective payment system (PPS) in such a way as to maximize income by giving as the principal diagnosis the one which places the patient in the highest-priced diagnosis related group (DRG), even though a lower-priced one more accurately reflects the patient's problem and the services rendered.

gap fill – A type of coverage particularly referencing Medicare where the benefits provided cover the deductibles and copays not paid by Medicare.

gastroenterology – The treatment of diseases and functions of the esophagus, stomach, and intestines; a subspecialty of internal medicine.

gatekeeper – A primary care provider or other individual who serves as a patient's initial contact for medical care and referrals. The gatekeeper acts as overall care coordinator, controlling a patient's access to specialty care referral or hospital admission by preauthorizing the visit, unless it is an emergency. In some health care delivery systems the gatekeeper is often a case manager or, in the case of behavioral health systems, a psychologist. The gatekeeper is primarily used in HMO settings.

gatekeeping – The process by which a gatekeeper directly provides the primary patient care and coordinates all diagnostic testing and specialty referrals required for a patient's medical care.

general care floor – Any patient care unit in a hospital that is not designated as a step-down unit (intermediate care or telemetry), intensive care unit or critical care unit.

general office expenses (GOE) – Expenses necessary for all plan administrative activities exclusive of claims administration expenses.

G

general practitioner – Physicians who provide medical care to all age groups, as in family practice.

generic drug – The established or official name by which a drug is known as an isolated substance, regardless of its manufacturer. Each drug is licensed under a generic name and also may be given a brand name by its manufacturer. Generics are typically less expensive and sold under a common name for that drug (e.g., the brand name "Valium" is also available under the generic name "diazepam"). Also called generic equivalent.

GHAA – Group Health Association of America. *See* AAHP.

global budget – A limit (cap) on total health care spending for a given population. In hospital systems, global budgeting is a cost containment method where participating hospitals share one prospectively set budget and allocate each hospital's funds from that one budget. Also known as total budget.

global capitation – Financial arrangements where health care providers (physicians and hospitals) assume full risk for the costs of caring for an entire enrollee population. Capitation rates are higher from health care plans and insurance companies, and physicians and hospitals retain control over medical decision-making. The drawback to the providers is that they must maintain quality care while reducing costs. Care that is cost excessive is paid for by the providers, not the health care plans or insurance companies. Hence, the risk. *See capitation.*

global fee – A method for paying hospital and physician services in one all-inclusive payment. For example, in a surgical case, there would be one global fee for all pre- and post-operative care. Managed care organizations prefer contracts with hospitals that contain set global fees, which help avoid any "surprise" costs. Global fee = hospital costs + hospital profits + physician fees. *See global pricing.*

global payments – *See global fee.*

global pricing – An agreement made between a payer and a hospital/physician in which both the hospital and physician fees are packaged into a single price, called global fee. That is, one payment for hospital and physician services. Also called packaged pricing. *See global fee.*

global surgery – HCFA-designed major surgical package that describes a normal surgical procedure with no complications that includes all of the elements needed to perform the procedure.

G

GME – *See graduate medical education.*

grace period – The period following the date premiums are due, during which payment of the membership dues may still be made without penalty or suspension of coverage.

graduate medical education – Refers to the formal medical education and training undertaken by physicians after they have attained their M.D. or D.O. degree.

grandfather clause – A clause of law that permits continued eligibility for individuals or organizations receiving program benefits under the law despite a change in the law which would otherwise make them ineligible.

grievance procedures – The process by which an insured patient or participating provider can submit complaints and seek remedies. Grievance procedures generally include a due process provision which guarantees that all grievances are subject to a specified and uniform adjudication method.

gross charges per 1000 – An indicator calculated by taking the gross charges incurred by a specific group for a specific period of time, dividing it by the average number of covered members in that group during the same period, then multiplying the result by 1000. This is calculated in the aggregate and by modality of treatment; e.g., inpatient, residential, partial hospitalization and outpatient. Gross charges per 1000 is used to evaluate utilization management performance and is a key concept for providers.

gross costs per 1000 – An indicator calculated by taking the gross costs incurred for services received by a specific group for a specific period of time, dividing it by the average number of covered members or lives in that group during the same period, and multiplying the result by 1000. This is calculated in the aggregate and by modality of treatment, e.g., inpatient, residential, partial hospitalization and outpatient. Like gross charges per 1000, gross costs per 1000 is used to evaluate utilization management performance. It is also a key concept for providers because in a managed care environment, it is necessary to keep gross costs per 1000 below collections per 1000.

group – The employer, association or organization through which subscribers and dependents become entitled to benefit coverage.

group contract – A contract of insurance made with an employer or other entity that covers a group of persons identified as individuals

G

by reference to their relationship to the entity. The agreement specifies rates, performance covenants, relationships among parties, schedule of benefits, and other conditions. The term of the group contract is generally limited to 12 months, and may be renewed after that.

group conversion – Subscribers who leave a group through which they are enrolled are offered an option to take a non-group program and pay premiums directly to a health plan, with continuity of service and without evidence of good health.

group coverage – A contract (certificate) between a health plan and the certificate holder (employer) which covers all group members. The employer is the certificate holder and contracting party, and the members receive an identification card as evidence they are covered.

group enrollment agreement – The agreement between a health plan and a group sponsor wherein the latter agrees to act as the sponsor and intermediary for a group.

Group Health Association of America (GHAA) – *See American Association of Health Plans* (AAHP).

group insurance – A health insurance policy where groups of employees and their dependents are covered under a single contract, issued by their employer or other group entity.

group insurance number – *See group number.*

group leader – A member of a group responsible for administering the group's program.

group model HMO – An HMO that contracts with a single group of physicians to provide care for its members. The physicians are paid a negotiated rate per patient (capitation rate) to provide a specified range of services. The physician group is then responsible for compensating each individual physician, sharing profits and contracting with hospitals for care of their patients.

These physician practices are usually located in hospitals or clinic settings, and members are required to receive medical care from a group physician unless a referral is made outside the network. A group model HMO is a form of a closed panel health plan. Also known as a prepaid group practice plan, group practice prepayment plan and prepaid health care.

group name – The legal name under which a group is enrolled.

G

group number – The number assigned to each covered group to identify the employer or a specific group of insured parties. The number appears on membership cards. Also called group insurance number.

group practice – A formal association of three or more physicians or other health professionals with income pooled and redistributed to the members of the group according to some pre-arranged plan. The group shares overhead expenses, medical and other records, transcription services, equipment and administrative staff, and acts as one when dealing with outside entities — such as HMOs.

group practice prepayment plan – *See group model* HMO.

group practice without walls (GPWW) – *See group without walls.*

group rider – Benefit coverage selected by an employer group which is appended to the basic coverage plan and applied to all employees who elect the coverage.

group sponsor – An individual or organization that agrees to sponsor a group and pay the dues and service charges to a health plan. The group sponsor acts as an agent for the group and its members, and agrees to receive the certificate and any information from the health plan on behalf of the group members.

group without walls (GWW) – A formal business entity that combines independent physicians or medical practices into a centralized management and decision-making structure. Under the GWW arrangement, physicians continue to practice in their own offices, but share administrative, billing and purchasing costs. The combined group contracts with managed care companies as a single entity, rather than as solo practitioners or small groups. Sometimes called group practice without walls.

guaranteed eligibility – A defined period of time (3-6 months) that all patients enrolled in prepaid health programs are considered eligible for Medicaid, regardless of their actual eligibility for Medicaid. A state may apply to the Health Care Financing Administration (HCFA) for a waiver to incorporate this into its contracts.

guaranteed issue – Requirement that health plans offer coverage to all businesses during some period each year.

guidelines – Statements by authoritative bodies (e.g., American College of Cardiology, American Academy of Pediatrics, etc.) as to the procedures appropriate for the physician to employ in making a diagnosis and treating it. The goal of guidelines is to change prac-

G

tice styles, reduce inappropriate and unnecessary care and cut costs.   Guidelines may also be referred to as practice parameters, clinical practice guidelines, clinical protocols and several other terms depending on the region of the country, medical school attended, provider experience, etc. In some ways, guidelines may be thought of as more general while protocols are more specific.

GWW – *See group without walls.*

gynecology – The diagnosis and treatment of diseases and disorders of the female reproductive system. In some health plans, gynecologists also act as primary care physicians, overseeing the general health of their patients.

handicapped dependent – The definition varies from plan to plan, but generally means unmarried dependent children who are incapable of self-support because of a physical or mental disability.

HCPP – *See health care prepayment plan.*

HCFA – *See Health Care Financing Administration.*

HCFA 1500 claim form – The mandatory claim form to be used for filing professional services with the nation's Medicare Part B and Medicaid carriers. HCFA's standard form for submitting physician service claims to third party (insurance) companies.

HCFA common procedural coding system (HCPCS) – Pronounced "hick picks." A system of codes and descriptive terminology used for reporting the provision of supplies, services and procedures to Medicare. It is a three-level coding system developed by HCFA and consisting of CPT codes, national alpha-numeric codes and local alpha-numeric codes. The alpha-numeric codes are for durable medical equipment, supplies, some drug items and special services. HCPCS codes are 5 digits, the first digit a letter followed by four numbers. Codes beginning with A through V are national; those beginning with W through Z are local. HCPCS is sometimes called health care procedural coding system.

HCPCS – *See HCFA common procedural coding system.*

health – The state of complete physical, mental and social well-being and not merely the absence of disease or infirmity. Most attempts at measuring health have been in terms of morbidity and mortality.

health alliances – *See health insurance purchasing cooperatives.*

Health and Human Services, The Department of (HHS) – The U.S. department responsible for health-related programs and issues. Formerly called HEW (Department of Health, Education, and Welfare).

health benefits package – *See benefit package.*

health care coalitions – A joint program usually involving health care providers, purchasers of care, industry, labor, and insurers in an attempt to deal with health care costs, issues and problems.

health care delivery – Loosely defined as providing any and all health care services to a population or community.

H

health care delivery system – Refers to all the facilities and services, as well as the methods for financing them, through which health care is provided.

Health Care Financing Administration (HCFA) – The government agency within the Department of Health and Human Services that administers the Medicare and Medicaid programs, and is responsible for overseeing Medicare and Medicaid payment regulations and the peer review organization (PRO).

Healthcare Integrity and Protection Data Bank (HIPDB) – A national health care fraud and abuse data collection program for reporting and disclosing certain final adverse actions taken against health care providers, suppliers, or practitioners. The HIPDB was created by the Health Insurance Portability and Accountability Act of 1996 (HIPAA).

Health care fraud burdens the nation with enormous financial costs and threatens the quality of health care and patient safety. Estimates of annual losses due to health care fraud range from 3 to 10 percent of all health care expenditures, which means it's in the billions of dollars. The HIPDB is related to and used in conjunction with the national practitioner data bank (NPDB). *See national practitioner data bank* (NPDB).

Health Care Organization (HCO) – A designation from the State of California for a formally organized managed care program for workers' compensation. California enacted the program in 1993 as part of a package of legislative reforms. The program specifies eligibility requirements, guidelines for physician choice, reimbursement methods, relationships with group health providers and length of medical control.

health care prepayment plan (HCPP) – A cost contract with the Health Care Financing Administration that prepays a health plan a flat amount per month to provide Medicare-eligible Part B medical services to enrolled members. Members pay premiums to cover the Medicare coinsurance, deductibles and copayments, plus any additional non-Medicare covered services that the plan provides. The HCPP does not arrange for Part A services.

Health Care Quality Improvement Act (HCQIA) – A 1996 federal act that: 1) provided liability protection for physicians and hospitals who participate in peer review, and 2) established a national clearinghouse to collect physician disciplinary and malpractice information.

H

health care professional – An individual who has received special training or education in a health-related field, including administration, direct provision of patient care or ancillary services. The professional may be licensed, certified or registered by a government agency or professional organization to provide specific health services in that field as an independent practitioner, or may be an employee of a healthcare facility.

health care provider – Anyone who delivers medical care or health care, including a doctor, hospital, laboratory or nurse.

health care reform – Refers to the attempts by Congress to "fix" the ails of the health care system, including the high costs of care, the lack of equal access for all Americans, and the overall inefficiencies in the system. Since the 1930s, the government has attempted to enact various legislation to constrain costs, increase accessibility and establish a national health program.

health care services plan – Any health care plan where a health insurance company or managed care organization contracts with health care providers to offer hospital and medical services to the health plan members on a prepaid basis. *See prepaid health care and prepaid health plan.*

health fair – An approach to offering health promotion services for self-referred participants who are encouraged to select the information and services of personal interest. Health fairs often include health information and education opportunities and some diagnostic screening, lifestyle assessment and counseling services directed at preventing disease and promoting health. Health fairs are usually community-based and may be targeted to a specific segment of the population.

health insurance – Coverage which provides payment of benefits for covered sickness or injury. Included under this heading are various types of insurance such as accident insurance, disability income insurance, medical expenses insurance, and accidental death and dismemberment insurance.

Health Insurance Portability and Accountability Act of 1996 (HIPAA) – Signed into law by President Bill Clinton on Aug. 21, 1996, this act limits exclusions for pre-existing medical conditions, prohibits discrimination against employees and dependents based on their health status, guarantees availability of health insurance to small employers, and guarantees renewability of insurance to all employers regardless of size. Portability means that individuals maintain their health coverage even though they switch employers or health plans.

H

health insurance purchasing cooperative (HIPC) – See *health plan purchasing cooperatives.*

health insuring organization (HIO) – An organization that contracts with a state or federal agency on a prepaid, capitated risk basis to provide comprehensive health services to beneficiaries of a state or federal program such as Medicaid or Medicare. The HIO, in turn, contracts with providers on a discounted FFS or a capitated basis to perform health services.

Health Level Seven (HL7) – An American National Standards Institute (ANSI) approved standard for electronic data exchange in health care that enables different computer applications to exchange clinical and administrative information. Since its protocols are flexible, HL7 has applicable CHIN (community health information network) use where data needs to be transmitted between institutions and systems. See *community health information network.*

Health Maintenance Act of 1990 – Originally developed by the National Association of Insurance Commissioners (NAIC), the Act has been used by most states as a model for legislation of Health Maintenance Organizations (HMOs). The act requires HMOs to have a certificate of authority to do business in the state and provide the state with detailed information, such as financials and quality data.

Health Maintenance Organization (HMO) – A health plan that delivers comprehensive, coordinated medical services to members on a pre-paid basis. HMOs focus on preventive medicine and managing care to keep health costs to a minimum. An HMO is paid monthly premiums or capitated rates by payers for each person enrolled, which is based on a projection of what the typical patient will cost. If enrollees cost more than the projection, the HMO could suffer losses. If the enrollees cost less, the HMO profits. This gives the HMO incentive to control costs. Payers include employers, insurance companies, government agencies, and other groups representing covered lives.

An HMO contracts with health care providers: physicians, hospitals, and other health professionals. HMO members are required to use participating or approved providers for all health services, and generally, all services will need to meet further approval by the HMO through its utilization program. Members select a primary care physician (PCP) from the HMO's list of affiliated doctors, and the PCP coordinates the patient's total care. When using medical services, members pay a small co-payment, but don't need to worry

H

about deductibles or claim forms.

HMOs may turn around and sub-capitate to other groups. For example, they may carve-out certain benefit categories, such as mental health, and subcapitate these to a mental health HMO; or they may subcapitate to a provider, provider group or provider network. HMOs are the most restrictive form of managed care benefit plans because they restrict the procedures, providers and benefits.

Under the Federal HMO Act, an entity must have three characteristics to call itself an HMO: 1) an organized system for providing health care or otherwise assuring health care delivery in a geographic area; 2) an agreed upon set of basic and supplemental health maintenance and treatment services; and 3) a voluntarily enrolled group of people. HMOs must also meet many rules and regulations required at the state level.

The four basic types of HMOs include:

* *Staff Model*—The HMO delivers services through providers who are salaried employees of the HMO.
* *Individual Practice Association* (IPA)—The HMO contracts with an organized group of physicians who come together for contracting purposes but retain their individual practices. The IPA physicians provide care to HMO members from their private offices and continue to see their fee-for-service patients.
* *Group* HMO—The HMO contracts with a multi-specialty medical group to provide care for HMO members, and the providers usually agree to devote a fixed percentage of time to the HMO.
* *Network model*—Similar to a Group HMO, but the HMO contracts for services with two or more medical groups.

Other types of HMOs include:

* *Direct Contract Model*—The HMO contracts directly with individual physicians.
* *Mixed Model*—The HMO gives members options that range from staff to IPA models.

Health Maintenance Organization Regulatory Agency – The state agency that oversees and licenses Health Maintenance Organizations (HMOs), and regulates its affairs in the best interest of consumers. In nearly all states, the HMO Regulatory Agency is the state insurance department.

health management – *See preventive care.*

H

Health Manpower Shortage Area (HMSA) – An area or group which the U.S. Department of Health and Human Services designates as having an inadequate supply of health care providers. HMSAs can include: (1) an urban or rural geographic area, (2) a population group for which access barriers can be demonstrated to prevent members of the group from using local providers, or (3) medium and maximum-security correctional institutions and public or non-profit private residential facilities.

health plan – Refers to the specific benefit package offered by an insurer; for example, the "HealthyChoice HMO" or the "TeamCare PPO." Also used to refer to the managed care or insurance company itself.

health plan document – *See plan document.*

Health Plan Employer Data and Information Set (HEDIS) – A core set of performance measures developed by National Committee on Quality Assurance (NCQA) to assist employers and other health purchasers in assessing health plan performance. HEDIS standardizes the way health plans report data in five major areas of health plan performance: quality, access and patient satisfaction, membership and utilization, finance, and descriptive information on health plan management.

health plan purchasing cooperatives (HPPC) – A health care purchasing entity formed by large groups of employers in a market for the purpose of shopping for health care on the basis of quality and the best price. HPPCs increase small employers' purchasing power by combining them with other companies and give them an incentive to provide health care to their employees. The intent of HPPCs is to leverage the combined employers' purchasing power to ensure that health care is delivered in economic and equitable ways. Also referred to as health insurance purchasing cooperatives, health insurance purchasing corporations, health alliances or regional health alliances.

health professional shortage areas (HPSA) – Federal designation for areas (counties, municipalities, etc.) with shortages of health care providers based on a population per physician ratio.

health promotion – Any combination of health information, education, diagnostic screening and healthcare interventions designed to facilitate behavioral alterations that will improve or protect health. It includes those activities intended to influence and support individual lifestyle modification and self-care.

health service agreement (HSA) – The detailed procedure and bene-

H

fit description given to each enrolled group. The HSA is the basis for discussion and explanation between the group and the health plan on issues related to enrollment, eligibility limitations, benefit descriptions, etc. *See contract.*

health services – Services intended to directly or indirectly contribute to the health and well-being of patients.

health services area – *See Health Systems Agency* (HSA).

health statement – A form which applicants complete attesting to their own and their dependents' health in order to secure membership.

health status – The measurement of a specific individual's or population's health based on their own subjective assessment of their health; by the incidence or prevalence of disease; or through mortality and morbidity data. Health status should be the measurement for effective health care, although sometimes it's difficult to separate the results of health care treatments from other factors that affect a patient's well being. *See outcomes and outcome research.*

health systems agency (HSA) – A health planning and resource development agency funded by the federal government and the states. HSAs are usually designated by a state to provide such services as health planning, monitoring, education and information for the population of a designated area (e.g., a state, a region within a state, etc.).

HEDIS – *See Health Plan Employer Data and Information Set. Also NCQA.*

hematology/oncology – Branch of internal medicine dealing with the treatment of diseases and disorders of the blood and blood-forming tissues, and the diagnosis and treatment of tumors and cancer.

HFMA – Healthcare Financial Management Association.

HHA – *See home health agency.*

HHS – *See health and human services.*

HIAA – Health Insurance Association of America.

HIC – Health insurance claim.

high-risk insurance pools – State programs that enable people with health problems to join together to purchase health insurance. Even with government subsidies, premium rates are high because pool members are high risk.

Hill-Burton Act – The 1946 federal law that provided grants and loans

H

to hospitals to upgrade and build new facilities in exchange for the hospitals' commitment to provide free or discounted prices for services rendered. The intent was to increase the number of hospital beds in poor or underserved communities of the United States. The Department of Health and Human Services (HHS) issued regulations that established standards for uncompensated care and specified that care provided to Medicare and Medicaid patients was not considered uncompensated care.

HIO – *See health insuring organization.*

HIPAA – *See Health Insurance Portability and Accountability Act of 1996.*

HIPC – Health insurance purchasing cooperative. *See health plan purchasing cooperative.*

HIPDB – *See Healthcare Integrity and Protection Data Bank.*

HL7 – *See Health Level Seven (HL7).*

HMO – *See Health Maintenance Organization.*

HMO Act of 1973 – Federal legislation which facilitated the growth and development of HMOs by providing HMO definitional requirements, federal grants and loans for HMO development and legislative mandates for HMO growth where previously prohibited.

HMO regulatory agency – *See Health Maintenance Organization Regulatory Agency.*

hold harmless clause – A clause frequently found in managed care contracts stating that if either the HMO or physician is held liable for malpractice, the other party is not. Hold harmless is also used in managed care contracts with providers that prohibit "balance billing" to health plan members for any covered benefit services other than deductibles, co-pays, and co-insurance. As such, the clause may be intended to prevent the provider from billing patients if their managed care company becomes insolvent.

The hold harmless clause relates primarily to UCR (usual, customary and reasonable) allowances, but has legal meaning as well. When applicable, "hold harmless" means that the managed care organization will assure that the patient will not be liable for any charges in excess of the UCR allowance.

holistic health – Emphasizes the well-being of every aspect of what makes a person whole and complete.

holistic medicine – Emphasizes treating the individual as a whole person.

H

home and community care for the functionally disabled – Defined under Section 1929 of the Social Security Act, which allows states to provide a broad range of home and community care to functionally disabled individuals as an optional state plan benefit. In all states but Texas the option can serve only people over 65. In Texas, individuals of any age may qualify to receive personal care services through section 1929 if they meet the state's functional disability test and financial eligibility criteria. Also known as the "frail elderly" provision.

home-based waiver – *See Section 1115(a).*

home care – Health care service(s) performed or supplied in the home of the patient.

home care program – A program through which a blend of health and social services are provided to individuals and families in their places of residence for the purpose of promoting, maintaining or restoring health or of minimizing the effects of illness and disability.

home health agency (HHA) – An agency that provides skilled nursing and other home health care services in the participant's home, and which is responsible for supervising the delivery of those services under a plan prescribed and approved in writing by the patient's physician. Home health care agencies must be licensed, certified or authorized pursuant to state and federal laws to provide such services.

home health care – The full range of medical and other health-related services such as physical and rehabilitation therapy, nursing, counseling and social services that are delivered in the home of a patient, by a provider. Home health care services are given to aged, disabled, sick or convalescent individuals who do not need institutional care. Home health agencies, hospitals and other community organizations provide these services.

home health care agency – *See home health agency.*

home health visit – Personal contact in the place of residence of a participant for the purpose of providing a covered service by a professional health worker.

homeopathy – A system of medicine based on the theory that diseases should be fought (1) by giving drugs that, in healthy persons, can produce the same symptoms from which the patient is suffering, and (2) by giving these drugs in minute doses. Compare to allopathy.

H

horizontal integration – Mergers between health care organizations that are at the same level in providing health care services. For example, mergers between hospital or hospitals and outpatient clinics. Compare to vertical integration. *See integrated delivery systems.*

hospice – A special kind of care for the dying and their families that treats the patient's medical, emotional and spiritual needs. Hospices emphasize alleviating pain and helping the patient and family make the most of the time left.

hospice care – Humane and supportive care services provided to a patient who is terminally ill and has a life expectancy of six months or less, and to the patient's family. The purpose of the services is to provide care for the patient without attempting to prolong his or her life.

hospice provider – A hospital, home health care agency or other provider which may legally render hospice care.

hospice services – *See hospice care.*

hospital – A health treatment facility capable of providing inpatient care that is appropriately staffed and equipped to provide diagnostic, therapeutic and preventive medical services. It must be duly licensed and operated as a hospital according to the laws of the state in which it is located. In the strictest definition, a convalescent, nursing, rest or extended care facility is not considered a hospital.

hospital, accredited – Hospital recognized upon inspection by the Joint Commission on Accreditation of Healthcare Organizations (JCAHO) as meeting its standards for quality of care, for the safety and maintenance of the physical plant, and for organization, administration and governance.

hospital affiliation – Refers to a contractual agreement between a health plan and one or more hospitals whereby the hospital provides the inpatient benefits offered by the health plan.

hospital alliances – Groups of hospitals that have joined together to share services and develop group purchasing programs to reduce their costs. *See also integrated delivery system, network and physician/hospital organization.*

hospital audit companies – Companies that provide retrospective audit services to hospitals in an attempt to achieve some percentage of savings from billed claims.

H

hospital care – Both in-patient and out-patient medical care which is provided and billed for by a hospital. Such care is subject to the rules and regulations of the hospital selected by the individual, and includes only the care acceptable to such hospital.

hospital confinement – A continuous period of inpatient hospital care.

hospital contract – The legal agreement between a health plan and a hospital covering the provision of care for members by a hospital and payment for such care by the plan.

hospital day – A 24-hour period when a patient is admitted to a hospital and receives hospital services. It is not considered a hospital day if the patient does not stay overnight or receives care on an outpatient basis. For hospital stays exceeding 24 hours, the day of admission is considered a hospital day; the day of discharge is not.

hospital days per 1000 – A measurement of the number of days of hospital care HMO members use in a year. It is calculated as follows: total number of days spent in a hospital by members divided by total members. This information is available through the Department of Health and Human Services and other sources.

hospital indemnity – A form of health insurance which provides a stipulated daily, weekly or monthly indemnity during hospital confinement. The indemnity is payable on an unallocated basis without regard to the actual expense of hospital confinement.

hospital number – The number assigned by a health plan to each member hospital for identification.

hospital savings – Savings accruing to a health plan due to contractual agreement between the plan and the member hospitals.

hospital services – Inpatient or outpatient care, procedures, supplies and services rendered to a patient by a hospital.

hospital-based physician – Physicians who spend the predominant part of their practice time within hospitals instead of in an office setting.

hospitalist – A physician who practices exclusively in hospitals or facilities, has no outpatient responsibilities, but works in all inpatient settings including acute, sub-acute and long-term care.

HPPC – *See health plan purchasing cooperatives.*

HPSA – *See Health Professional Shortage Area.*

HSA – Health service agreement. *See contract.*

HSA – *See Health System Agency.*

IBNR – *See incurred but not reported.*

ICD-9-CM – *See International Classification of Diseases, 9th Edition, Clinical Modification.*

ICD-10-CM – *See International Classification of Diseases, 10th Edition, Clinical Modification.*

ICF MR (intermediate care facility for mentally retarded persons) – Optional Medicaid service which provides residential care and services for individuals with developmental disabilities. Each state defines the levels of ICF MR care. *See intermediate care facility.*

ICU – *See intensive care unit.*

identification card (ID card) – The card issued to a health plan subscriber as evidence of proof of membership, showing name, number, and types of coverage. This card must be displayed by participants to providers when care is obtained. Also called membership card.

identification number (ID #) – A number that appears on the health plan identification card and is used on all claims, communications and inquiries. In some cases, the identification number is the same as the subscriber's social security number.

IDS – *See integrated delivery system.*

IME – *See independent medical evaluation.*

immediate annuity – An annuity that begins making periodic payments to the annuitant within one year from date of purchase.

immediate non-emergency care – Medical, surgical or dental care for other than an emergency condition, which is necessary at the time and place for the health and well being of the member.

impact program – A cost management program that encourages wise use of health care services and benefits. It controls expensive inpatient hospital care, shifting treatment to less expensive settings when appropriate and making sure patients do not spend more time than necessary in the hospital.

in-before-service – This term means a patient receives services prior to the effective date of membership in a health plan.

inactive – Refers to the status of a group or subscriber relating to their

I

health insurance. Inactive means that the health insurance has been canceled or is no longer effective.

incentives – Financial motivators given to providers to promote efficiency and quality in health care delivery. The incentives are profit-sharing arrangements offered by managed care plans that permit subcontractors and physicians to share in amounts earned from plan savings through reduced hospital and specialty referral usage. Incentives are used to encourage physicians to decrease hospital days, increase preventive health care, consider alternative treatments, etc.

incentivize – Not a real term found in a dictionary, but widely used throughout managed care meaning a way to motivate providers through the use of incentives. Usage: "Managed care organizations continuously look for ways to incentivize physicians to provide quality care at the best cost."

incidence – The frequency of occurrence of disease, infection or some other event measured in terms of a population. For example, the number of cases of chicken pox occurring in a school during a month in relation to the number of children in the school. Compare to prevalence (the number of cases of a disease, etc.).

incur – To become liable for a loss, claim or expense. Cases or losses incurred are those occurring within a fixed period for which an insurance plan becomes liable whether or not reported, adjusted, and paid.

incurred but not reported (IBNR) – A cash reserve set up by a payer (managed care company or health insurer) to cover costs associated with a medical service that has been provided, but for which a claim has not yet been received by the payer. The IBNR cash reserves are an estimate of the claims that are the responsibility of the health plan, based on studies of prior lags in claim submissions.

incurred claims – The dollar amount of claims attributable to a particular period of time, regardless of when those claims are actually paid.

incurred claims loss ratio – The ratio of claims incurred to premiums earned. That is, incurred claims plus expenses, divided by premiums.

incurred-to-paid ratios – Factors to adjust annual paid claims to annual incurred claims.

indemnify – An insurance term meaning "to compensate for a loss."

I

indemnity – A benefit paid by an insurance policy for an insured loss. Often it is used to refer to benefits paid directly to the insured in a pre-determined amount for covered expenses.

indemnity carrier – Usually an insurance company or insurance group that agrees to assume health insurance risk for its subscribers at some pre-determined rate. Insured individuals are reimbursed after carriers review and process filed claims. All costs above the fixed insurance payment are the patient's responsibility. *See indemnity plan.*

indemnity insurance – *See indemnity plan.*

indemnity plan – A type of insurance plan under which individuals pay 100% of all medical bills up to an annual deductible. The insurance company then pays a percentage of all covered charges up to an out-of-pocket maximum. Indemnity plans offer virtually unlimited choice of physicians and hospitals, but at a higher cost than managed care plans. Coverage is usually limited to a percentage of the billed amount, and providers are reimbursed each time they provide a service; that is, on a fee-for-service basis. Indemnity plans are the opposite of managed care plans with no imposing quality or cost-control measures; patients have free choice and providers can bill without restrictions. Sometimes referred to as a traditional insurance plan. *See also fee-for-service.*

independent medical evaluation (IME) – An examination carried out by an impartial health care provider for the purpose of resolving a dispute related to the nature and extent of an illness or injury.

Independent Physician Association (IPA) – *See Individual Practice Association.*

Independent Practice Association (IPA) – *See Individual Practice Association.*

indirect insurance payments – Payments sent to the patient as reimbursement for medical expenses incurred and paid.

individual consideration – A claim that has to be specially reviewed because an established allowance or benefit determination has not been made due to the uniqueness or variance in the service rendered.

individual deductible – Amount of covered expenses that an individual participant must incur and be responsible to pay before a health plan will make payment for membership benefits.

I

individual membership – One person or single membership as opposed to "family membership."

individual plan – A type of insurance plan for individuals and their dependents who are not eligible for medical insurance under a group policy (group coverage). Sometimes called personal insurance, as distinct from group and blanket insurance.

Individual Practice Association (IPA) – An HMO model in which the health plan contracts with an organized group of physicians who come together for contracting purposes while retaining their individual practices. The IPA physicians provide care to HMO members from their private offices and continue to see their fee-for-service patients. Depending on the IPA, physicians are compensated on a per capita fee schedule, or fee-for-service basis. Also known as Independent Practice Association or Independent Physician Association. This type of system combines prepayment with the traditional means of delivering health care.

individual specific stop loss – If a member of a group incurs claims in excess of a specified dollar limit during a contract period, the excess amount is not charged against the group's experience. *See stop loss.*

infectious diseases – Medical diagnosis and treatment of acute and chronic infections.

infertility – Branch of medicine which determines cause and treatment of the inability to conceive.

informed consent – Refers to the premise that no treatment or procedure will be performed, or medication given without the consent of the patient while he or she has the capacity to understand the information being given. Additionally, it holds that patients have the right to know what their choices are and the risks that are associated with such choices.

inlier – A patient whose length of stay or treatment cost resembles those of most other patients in a diagnosis-related group.

in-network – A group of doctors, hospitals and other health care providers who contract with a health plan to provide care for plan members at special rates and to handle the paperwork with the health plan.

inpatient (IP) – A person who receives care as a registered bed-patient for a minimum of 24 hours and is charged a daily room and board fee.

I

inpatient benefits – Refers to the benefits an individual is covered for as an inpatient. Inpatient benefits usually include charges for room and board and charges for necessary services and supplies (sometimes referred to as hospital extras, miscellaneous charges, and ancillary charges).

inpatient care – Care given to a registered bed-patient in a hospital, nursing home or other medical or post-acute care institution.

inpatient hospital claim – A request for payment of benefits for bed-patient services incurred by a member at a recognized hospital.

inpatient hospital stay – The time from the day of admission to the day of discharge of a bed-patient. Includes the day of admission but not the day of discharge in the length of stay calculations.

inpatient services – Inpatient hospital services are items and services furnished to an inpatient of a hospital by the hospital. Inpatient services include bed and board, nursing and related services, diagnostic and therapeutic services, and medical or surgical services.

inside limit – A maximum limitation placed on the payment for a particular benefit included in the coverage for that type of expense. For example, $100 limit on hospital room and board.

insolvency – A legal determination occurring when a managed care plan no longer has the financial reserves or other arrangements to meet its contractual obligations to patients and subcontractors.

installment settlement – Payment of the policies' proceeds in installments rather than in a lump sum.

institutional providers – Refers to hospitals, nursing homes, day care centers, alcohol and substance abuse centers, etc., as opposed to individual providers such as physicians, dentists, chiropractors, etc.

instrumental Activities of Daily Living – Refers to a person's ability to perform activities that are necessary for living independently in the community, such as preparing meals, shopping for routine items, managing money and housekeeping. Compare to Activities of Daily Living (ADL).

insurable risk – Refers to the potential of a risk to be insured. The conditions that make a risk insurable are: a) it must produce a definite loss not under the control of the insured; b) there must be others subject to the same risks; c) the loss must be measurable and the cost of insuring it must be financially viable; d) the risk must be unlikely to affect all insured simultaneously; e) the loss must have

I

a potential to be financially serious.

insurance – Protection against risk or loss whereby one party contracts to guarantee another party, in return for the payment of a premium, against financial loss in the event of some contingency or peril.

insurance carrier – The insurance company that sells the policies and administers the contract. Also called the insurer.

insurance department – Each state government has an insurance department that is responsible for implementing state insurance laws and regulations.

insured – The person who contracts with an insurance company for insurance coverage. Sometimes called a policyholder or subscriber.

integrated delivery system (IDS) – A health care provider organization that combines physicians, hospitals and other medical services to deliver coordinated, continuing ambulatory and tertiary care to the population and to managed care organizations. As one fully integrated health care entity, it has the ability to strongly negotiate with managed care organizations. The most advanced IDS form includes an insurance or TPA (third party administrator) function to eliminate the division between provider and payer.

Integrated delivery systems utilize both horizontal integration and vertical integration for growing their networks and services. This "network of organizations" provides a coordinated continuum of health care to the community, offering full health care services and improving the health status of individuals. Consequently, it is accountable for the outcomes of the populations served. Also called integrated medical system (IMS), integrated healthcare system (IHS), integrated health system (IHS), integrated healthcare organization (IHO), integrated health delivery system (IHDS) and integrated service network (ISN). *See Accountable Health Plan (AHP) and Outcomes.*

integrated healthcare system (IHS) – *See integrated delivery system.*

integrated health delivery system (IHDS) – *See integrated delivery system.*

integrated healthcare organization (IHO) – *See integrated delivery system.*

integrated health system (IHS) – *See integrated delivery system.*

integrated medical system (IMS) – *See integrated delivery system.*

integrated provider network (IPN) – Comprised of primary and secondary hospitals and providers within a geographical area.

I

integrated service network (ISN) – *See integrated delivery system* (IHS).

integration – Describes when providers (hospitals, physicians, etc.) combine operations in an attempt to cut costs and increase health care services and productivity. There are different levels of integration from simple coordination (e.g., consolidated purchasing) to full integration (e.g., centralized administration and consolidated care coordination).

integrative medicine – Refers to the combination of conventional and alternative medicine in the treatment of patients. Some medical researchers and physicians believe that integrative medicine best addresses a patient's physical, mental and emotional needs.

intensive care – Care rendered to patients who are unable to maintain vital functions, require immediate and continuous nursing care, and may not be able to communicate their needs. Patients often have complex medical problems. Examples include patients with massive hemorrhage, neurosurgical, orthopedic, vascular, or burn injuries; post-surgical patients; and patients with infectious diseases, malaria, fever of unknown origin, and gastrointestinal conditions such as ulcers and dysentery. Various life support systems such as respirators, monitors, pumps and hypothermia equipment are standard items used in this setting.

intensive care unit (ICU) – A unit in the hospital in which a patient receives an intensive level of care. Special life-saving techniques and equipment are regularly and immediately available, and patients are under continuous observation by a nursing staff specially trained and selected. There can be several ICUs within a hospital, including the medical intensive care unit (MICU), the surgical intensive care unit (SICU), the pediatric intensive care unit (PICU), the neonatal intensive care unit (NICU), and the coronary care unit (CCU). Sometimes called special care unit.

intensivist – A physician who specializes in critical care.

intergovernmental initiative (IGI) – Cooperative arrangement between local government entities in which local dollars used for indigent care are contributed as a match to draw down federal Medicaid dollars. IGIs are responsible for management of the delivery system.

intermediary – Blue Cross and Blue Shield Plans and commercial insurance companies which hold contracts with the Social Security Administration to administer the Part A program of the Medicare program.

I

intermediate care – Care rendered to patients who require observation and nursing care at a less intense level than the provided in the intensive care unit (ICU), but more than would be applied on a general care floor. Intermediate care is provided in a step-down unit (sometimes called an intermediate care unit) for patients that don't need the intensive services of an acute hospital setting, but are not ready to be released to independent care at home. Sometimes called subacute care. *See step-down unit and intensive care.*

intermediate care facility (ICF) – Refers to a facility that provides a level of care that is less than the degree of care and treatment that a hospital or skilled nursing facility is designed to provide, but at a greater level than just room and board.

internal medicine – Diagnosis and non-surgical treatment of diseases and disorders of adults. Specifically, internal medicine refers to the study and treatment of internal organs and body systems, and encompasses many subspecialties.

International Classification of Diseases, 9th Edition, Clinical Modification (ICD-9-CM) – *See International Classification of Diseases, 10th Edition, Clinical Modification (ICD-10-CM).*

International Classification of Diseases, 10th Edition, Clinical Modification (ICD-10-CM) – A listing of diagnoses and identifying codes used by physicians for reporting the incidence of disease, injury, mortality and illness. The coding and terminology provide a uniform language that can accurately designate primary and secondary diagnoses and provide for reliable, consistent communication on claim forms. Developed by the World Health Organization, the ICD has been revised periodically to incorporate changes in the medical field. To date, there have been 10 revisions of the ICD since the year 1900. The 10th edition was introduced in 1999.

intervention strategy – A generic term used in public health to describe a program or policy designed to have an impact on an illness or disease. For example, a mandatory seat belt law is an intervention strategy designed to reduce automobile-related fatalities.

IP – Abbreviation for inpatient. *See inpatient.*

IPA – *See Individual Practice Association.*

IPP – *See individual practice program.*

ISN – Integrated service network.

itemized bill – A bill or invoice indicating patient's name, provider's name, date of each service, type of service and the charge for each.

JCAHO – *See Joint Commission on Accreditation of Healthcare Organizations.*

job-lock – Individuals' inability to change jobs because they would lose crucial health benefits.

Joint Commission on Accreditation of Health Care Organizations (JCAHO) – A private, not-for-profit organization that evaluates and accredits hospitals and other health care organizations providing home care, mental health care, ambulatory care, and long term care services. JCAHO was established in 1951 to enhance the quality of care provided by hospitals and other organizations by monitoring and implementing standards of practice that organizations must achieve to receive recognition and accreditation. JCAHO revises its standards every year, but reviews organizations approximately every 3 years. These reviews involve JCAHO medical and administrative representatives who analyze the organization's policies, patient records, credentialing procedures and quality assurance programs.

Julian date – Actual number of the day within the year (i.e., January 31, 1998 is Julian date 98031).

jumbo claim – *See large claim.*

Katie Beckett option – *See* TEFRA 134(*a*).

knowledge-based system – A computer system that uses stored expert knowledge to support health care providers in making clinical decisions and solving problems.

Knox-Keene Act – California legislation (1975) amending the Health and Safety Code that licenses HMOs separately from insurance companies. Provides for regulation by the Commissioner of Corporations.

L

lapse – Termination of a policy upon the policyholder's failure to pay the premium within the time required.

large claim – The sum of covered medical expenses of a member which exceeds a specified claim limit. Typical limits range from $25,000 to $50,000 with amounts as high as $100,000. Also called jumbo claim or shock claim.

large claim pooling – A system that isolates claims above a certain dollar level and charges them to a pool funded by the charges of all groups who share the pool. Large claim pooling is designed to help stabilize significant premium fluctuations. *See risk pool.*

large groups – Depends on each state, but usually defined as groups with 100 or more eligible employees.

large group health plan – Employer-sponsored group health plan that covers 20 or more employees (this number varies between states) and is primary to Medicare.

left employment – Terminated employment at company. May be eligible for continuation of coverage with group or for direct pay coverage.

legend drug – Drug that the law says can only be obtained by prescription. *See also formulary and drug formulary.*

length of stay – The total number of days that a covered person stayed in an inpatient facility such as a hospital, extended care facility or skilled nursing facility.

lenses – Refers to any ophthalmic corrective lenses prescribed by a physician or optometrist to improve visual perception.

letter of intent – A letter of understanding sent to a physician who is salaried by an institution for services performed and also maintains a separate office for private practice.

liability –
  1. Any insurance claim that has not yet been paid or completed.
  2. The probable cost of meeting an obligation.

liability insurance – Insurance which reimburses the policyholder in the event someone is injured by the insured, by an object owned by the insured, or on the insured's premises. Malpractice, auto, and homeowners insurance are all specific types of liability insurance.

L

licensed beds – *See beds, licensed.*

licensed health care professional – A physician or other professional provider duly licensed to render care to patients.

licensed practical nurse (LPN) – A person duly licensed as a practical nurse (LPN) by the state in which such person is engaged in the practice of nursing (in California and Texas licensing is as an LVN or licensed vocational nurse). LPNs provide nursing care and treatment of patients under the supervision of a licensed physician or registered nurse.

licensed vocational nurse (LVN) – *See licensed practical nurse* (LPN) *and practical nurses.*

licensing – Describes the process most states employ to review and approve applications from Health Maintenance Organizations (HMOs) prior to beginning their operations in certain areas of the state. Areas examined by the licensing authority usually include the HMO's fiscal soundness, network capacity and quality assurance. The applicant must demonstrate it can meet all existing statutory and regulatory requirements prior to beginning operations.

life annuity – A contract that provides a stated income for life.

lifetime maximum – The maximum dollar amount that an insurance company will pay toward an insured's claims in a lifetime and/or the maximum dollar amount paid for all covered sicknesses and injuries for each insured person while the insurance certificate is in effect. Also called total certificate membership benefit maximum.

lifetime maximum benefit – *See lifetime maximum.*

lifetime reserve days – A Medicare term referring to the 60 days that Medicare provides for beneficiaries for payment of benefits beyond the maximum benefit days limit. The 60-day lifetime reserve is reduced by any additional days used by a Medicare beneficiary beyond their benefit exhausted date. *See benefit exhausted date.*

limitations – Limitations describe conditions or circumstances under which the insurer will not pay or will limit payments. Detailed information about limitations and exclusions is found in the certificate of insurance. An employer receives a group policy, with all details of the contract, while an employee receives a booklet with a more concise presentation of the insurance contract.

line of business (LOB) – Defines a classification of business for allocating both income and expenses. For example, underwritten hos-

L

pitalization coverage is one line of business and underwritten medical/surgical coverage is another.

LOB – *See line of business.*

locality – A specific geographic area within which Medicare carriers establish prevailing charges. Localities are unique for each Medicare carrier and the criteria for definition of the locality may be states, counties, population density, metropolitan size or other factor.

location – Where services are rendered — a doctor's office, clinic, inpatient and outpatient, etc.

location code (professional provider) – A numeric designation found on the provider file and on a claim form. If a provider practices at more than one address, each address is identified by its unique location code.

lock-in – A contractual provision by which members are required to receive all their care from the network health care providers, except in cases of urgent or emergency need. Primarily applies to Health Maintenance Organization (HMO) members.

long-term acute care (LTAC) – The Long Term Acute Care Hospital Association of America (LTACHAA) defines LTAC as providing specialized acute hospital care for medically complex patients who are critically ill, have multisystem complications and/or failures, and require hospitalization averaging 25 days. The goal in long-term acute care is medical recovery and return to home and family versus stabilization.

long-term care (LTC) – Assistance and care on a recurring or continuous basis for patients who require help with the Activities of Daily Living (ADLs) or who suffer from a cognitive impairment. LTC patients are those who are chronically ill, aged, disabled or retarded. Care is provided either in an institution or at home.

long-term care hospital (LTCH) – A Medicare term referring to a hospital with an average patient stay longer than 25 days, and not otherwise a rehabilitation or psychiatric hospital. Patients are transferred to these specialty hospitals because the severity and complexity of their medical conditions require extended treatment that would be inappropriate for admission into a nursing home or rehabilitation hospital.

Long-term care hospitals focus on patients with medically complex conditions or multiple conditions (comorbidities). Many of the

L

patients are admitted directly from a short-stay hospital intensive care unit (ICU) with respiratory or ventilator-dependent conditions or other complex medical conditions requiring intensive and continuous acute care services. Their clinical and therapeutic intervention usually involves daily physician visits, 24-hour RN care, significant ancillary services and complicated medication regimens. Also called long-term acute care hospital.

long term care insurance – Insurance designed to pay for some or all of the costs of long-term care.

long-term disability – When a non-occupational accident or sickness keeps an insured employee from performing the duties of his or her job for a long period of time.

long-term disability insurance – Insurance issued to an employer or individual to provide a reasonable replacement of a portion of an employee's earned income that may be lost because of serious and prolonged illness or injury during their normal work career. Also called long-term disability income insurance.

LOS – *See length of stay.*

loss ratio – *See incurred claims loss ratio and medical loss ratio.*

LTC – *See long term care.*

M

MAC – Maximum allowable cost. This term is most frequently used in connection with prescription drugs, and generally refers to the cost of a generic drug dispensed.

major diagnosis – The condition that consumes the most resources during a hospital stay. The major diagnosis may differ from the admitting and principal diagnoses.

major diagnostic categories (MDCs) – Twenty-three (23) broadly defined clinical categories that are based on body system, causes of disease, disease location, and signs and symptoms (*See* ICD-9-CM). The 23 MDCs subdivide into the diagnosis related groups (DRGs), and are commonly used for aggregated DRG reporting.

major medical – A health insurance plan designed to help offset the heavy medical expenses resulting from catastrophic or prolonged illness or injury. After a deductible is paid by the insured person, major medical insurance covers a wide range of medical care charges (typically 75-80%) with few internal limits and a high over-all maximum benefit. The major medical policy provides benefits for hospital, surgical and medical services, prescription drugs, durable medical equipment (DME), and private duty nursing. Sometimes called major medical expense insurance.

major medical expense insurance – *See major medical.*

maldistribution – The surplus or shortage of health providers needed to maintain the health status of a given population. Maldistribution can occur both geographically and by specialty. *See health professional shortage area* (HPSA).

malpractice – Professional misconduct or lack of ordinary skill in the performance of a professional act. A practitioner is liable for dam-ages or injuries caused by malpractice if the patient can prove some injury and that the injury was the result of negligence on the part of the professional.

malpractice insurance – Insurance against the risk of suffering finan-cial damage due to professional misconduct or lack of ordinary skill.

managed behavioral health program (MBHP) – A managed care pro-gram specifically for behavioral health care, usually under a "carve-out" arrangement by a managed care organization (MCO) or insurance company. That is, the MCO or insurance company con-tracts with a managed behavioral health company to provide serv-

M

ices to the health plan's members. The program may include providing behavioral services, utilization management services or organizing an employee assistance program (EAP). The program may be reimbursed on a sub-capitation, capitation or fee-for-service (FFS) basis. MBHPs are considered specialty MCOs. *See carve-out, managed care and managed care organization.*

managed care – A system that uses financial incentives and management controls to direct patients to providers who are responsible for giving appropriate, cost-effective care. Managed care is a fundamental shift in the health system from more expensive reactive care to care that is more proactive. As such, managed care systems are intended to control the cost of health care by emphasizing prevention, early intervention and outpatient care. A managed care system may include health insurers, medical groups, hospitals and health systems.

The term "managed care" was originally intended to refer to prepaid health plans, like HMOs, that assumed risk for a defined population. But over time, it has increasingly been used to describe health care that incorporates preadmission certification, case management, provider incentives, medically necessary reviews, and other utilization controls. It has been broadly used to describe types of organizations, payment mechanisms, review procedures, collaborations, and incentive plans.

Often times, managed care is used as a general term for the activity of organizing doctors, hospitals, and other providers into groups in order to enhance the quality and cost-effectiveness of health care. Organizations that engage in managed care (managed care organizations or MCOs) include HMOs, PPOs, POSs, EPOs, PHOs, IDSs, AHPs and IPAs. Many state Medicaid programs also include managed care components as a method of ensuring quality in a cost efficient manner.

The overall value of managed care is unknown, probably due to the fact that the term "managed care" has such diverse meanings depending on the health care entity using the term. Regardless of the definition one uses, the key question is whether managed care can effectively lower health care costs while building a more efficient health care system. Also called managed health care.

managed care organization (MCO) – A health plan that seeks to manage the care of its health plan members by combining health care financing and delivery. MCOs contract with providers to deliver care to its members, and providers are reimbursed utilizing various

M

methods, including capitation, sub-capitation, fee-for-service (FFS) or discounted FFS. Since they are accountable for the health of their members, MCOs seek to deliver quality care at the lowest cost possible using a wide range of managed care techniques; for example, utilization management (UM) and case management. Many MCOs utilize complex information systems that are capable of monitoring and evaluating trends of medical service usage and the cost of those services. A managed care organization can be an HMO, PPO, POS, EPO, PHO, IDS, AHP or IPA. *See managed care.*

managed competition – A health care system where employers form large alliances to buy health care coverage at a lower cost. The employers each make a specified contribution toward health care insurance for the employees in their group, and the employees would be responsible for selecting the health plan they prefer. Since the employees are responsible for the difference between the amount their employer contributes and the cost of the health plan, they have an incentive to be more price-conscious. At the same time, health care insurers are encouraged to hold down the cost of their plans to make them more competitive.

managed fee-for-service – A fee-for-service (FFS) payment system combined with some components of managed care. The cost of covered services is paid by the insurer after services have been received by the patient. Various managed care tools such as pre-certification, second surgical opinion, and utilization review are used.

managed health care – *See managed care.*

managed health care plan – *See managed care organization.*

managed indemnity plan – A fee-for-service (FFS) health plan that uses a limited number of managed care techniques such as utilization review in the form of pre-certification for hospital and outpatient services. *See pre-certification and utilization review.*

management services organization (MSO) – A legal entity that provides practice management, administrative and support services to individual physicians, hospitals or group practices. The MSO may own the facilities and employ the non-physician staff used to deliver care. Further, an MSO may be a direct subsidiary of a hospital or may be owned by investors. *See medical services organization.*

mandated benefits – Benefits that a health plan must provide by state or federal law. For example, some states have mandated 48-hour maternity stays following vaginal deliveries. *See also mandated or required services.*

M

mandated or required services – Services which a state is required to offer to needy individuals under a state Medicaid plan. Medically needy persons may be offered a more restrictive service package. Mandated services include:

- hospital (inpatient & outpatient)
- lab/x-ray
- nursing facility care (21 and over)
- home health care
- family planning
- physician
- nurse midwives
- dental (medical/surgical)
- rural health clinic
- certain nurse practitioners
- federally qualified health centers
- renal dialysis services
- EPSDT (under age 21)
- medical transportation

mandatory enrollment – Requirement that certain groups of people must enroll in a program. For example, Medicaid managed care.

mandated benefits – This term primarily relates to goods and services that must be covered for benefit payments as specified primarily under federal or state regulations. For example, a regulation that mandates that certain minimum benefits must be paid for alcoholism under all insurance contracts sold in the state.

mandated providers – Providers whose services must be included in coverage offered by a health plan. These mandates can be required by state or federal law.

mandated services – *See mandated benefits.*

manual rating – Refers to obtaining a rate by referencing a book or manuals that contain relative relationships among various types of benefits and incorporate age-sex, industry and area factors. These rates represent the expected costs of coverage for a particular group or class.

margin – Provision for error when making estimates of advance premium rates and reserve requirements.

market area – The targeted geographic areas where a health plan's main market potential is located. A health plan's market area is not necessarily the same as its service area, although they often overlap.

M

market segment – This term is used to identify a particular class, set or type of enrolled or potentially enrolled customer. For example, non-group participants who are not eligible for Medicare, groups under 200 employees, or ASO or self-funded groups may all be considered segments.

market share – That part of the market potential that a managed care company (e.g., HMO or fee-for-service/prepaid medical group) has captured; usually market share is expressed as a percentage of the market potential.

master contract – The legal agreement between a group and the health plan defining the terms and conditions of their program.

master patient/member index – An index or file with a unique identifier for each patient or member that serves as a key to a patient's or member's health record.

maternity care – Hospital care in obstetrical cases including the use of the delivery room, post-delivery care and nursery care of the newborn.

maturity factor – Factor to annualize claims where less than one year's experience is available. For example, if only 8 months of claims are available for analysis, the total dollar amount for those claims would be multiplied by a maturity factor of 1.5 to attain a one year claim amount ($8 \times 1.5 = 12$).

maximum allowable – The amount set by an insurance company as the highest amount that it will pay for a particular medical service or procedure. Actual payments by a third party may be less than the maximum allowable due to the member's deductibles and co-insurance. Also called maximum allowable charge, maximum allowable amount, allowed amount or approved amount.

maximum allowable actual charge (MAAC) – A limitation on billed charges for Medicare services provided by non-participating physicians.

maximum allowable cost list (MAC) – A PBM's (pharmacy benefit manager) or health plan's listing of the maximum price paid for a generic drug. For example, generic ampicillin 250mg capsules may be available from various manufacturers at a range of prices from 5 cents to 5 dollars per capsule. A PBM or health plan will decide how much they are willing to pay for this drug, usually a price near the low end of the scale. When they do so, they have assigned a "maximum allowable cost" to ampicillin 250mg capsules. They must do

M

the same thing for every other dosage form and strength of the drug.

The listing is distributed to participating pharmacies and is subject to periodic review by the PBM or health plan. Covered members have to pay a cost differential for a brand name version of their prescriptions.

maximum allowable cost program (MAC) –
1. A federal program that limits reimbursement for prescription drugs under the Medicaid programs. The MAC is the lowest unit price at which a drug available from several sources can be purchased on a national basis.
2. The administration and management of a pharmacy benefit manager's (PBM's) or health plan's maximum allowable cost list. *See maximum allowable cost list* (MAC).

maximum benefits – The highest amount the insurance company will pay for medical claims during a specified period. This amount is set either on a yearly basis or for the lifetime of the policy. *See lifetime maximum benefit.*

maximum claim liability – The maximum dollar amount of claims payment for which a group is liable.

maximum out-of-pocket – The maximum amount an employee has to pay in any year toward the cost of medical treatment; usually the total of the deductible and coinsurance amounts.

McCarran-Ferguson Act – A 1945 Act of Congress exempting insurance businesses from federal commerce laws and delegating regulatory authority to the states.

M+C – *See Medicare + Choice.*

MCO – Managed care organization.

MCPI – Medical Consumer Price Index (U.S. Dept. of Labor statistics).

MCR – Modified community rating.

M.D. – Doctor of Medicine.

Medicaid (Title XIX) – A federally-aided, state operated and administered program which provides medical benefits for certain persons whose income and resources are considered insufficient to pay for health care costs (i.e., poor, elderly and disabled). Each state, under broad federal guidelines, determines qualifying requirements, benefit level and amount of provider reimbursement. The program was enacted in 1965 under Title XIX of the Social Security Act.

M

medical assistant – An employee of a professional provider whose duties usually include securing insurance information from patients, filing insurance claims, billing and posting, and other clerical duties. Other activities may also include obtaining medical information, assisting with examinations, and other medical-related activities.

medical care – Care other than surgery and obstetrical services which Doctors of Medicine, Doctors of Osteopathy and other licensed health care professionals render to patients.

medical care evaluation studies (MCE) – A form of health care review in which problems in the quality of the delivery and organization of health care services are addressed and monitored.

medical cost ratio (MCR) – *See medical loss ratio.*

medical director – A physician, usually employed by a hospital or managed care organization, who serves in a medical and administrative capacity as liaison for the medical staff with the administration and governing body.

medical emergency – *See emergency.*

medical foundation – An organization of physicians, sometimes sponsored by a state or local medical association, that develops a management structure and administrative functions. Foundations usually operate as prepaid group practices or as an individual practice association (IPA), and market themselves to managed care organizations (e.g., HMOs). Even though their contracts with such organizations may be on a capitated basis, foundations pay their members on a fee-for-service (FFS) basis. Most foundations are organized for peer review purposes, but may also conduct utilization management. Also known as a foundation.

Medical Group Management Association (MGMA) – The MGMA is a national professional and trade association representing physician group practices. The association provides its members with extensive data on such areas as physician compensation, performance efficiency, and physician practice comparisons.

medical group practice – The American Group Practice Association (AGPS), the American Medical Association (AMA), and the Medical Group Management Association (MGMA) define medical group practice as: "provision of health care services by a group of at least three licensed physicians engaged in a formally organized and legally recognized entity sharing equipment, facilities, common

M

records and personnel involved in both patient care and business management."

medical informatics – The systematic science of the storage, retrieval, analysis and communication of clinical data to improve decisions made by physicians and managers of health care organizations.

medical information – Data required regarding the onset, history or extent of a particular illness or condition in order for a health plan to determine if benefits are available for current treatment for that condition.

medical insurance – A contract between the policyholder (insured) and an insurance company (insurer) for reimbursement of a portion of the policyholder's cost of medical treatment for a stated diagnosis.

medical IRAs – See *medical savings account* (MSA).

medical loss ratio (MLR) – The amount of revenues from health insurance premiums that is spent to pay for the medical services covered by the health plan. MLR is stated as a ratio as a percentage of premium revenues, such as 0.98, meaning that 98% of premiums were spent on purchasing medical services. Managed care and health insurance companies work to keep the MLR below 1.00, since their profit comes from premiums. Most HMOs try to maintain MLRs in the 0.70-0.80 range. *See also loss ratio and incurred claims loss ratio.* Sometimes called Medical Cost Ratio.

medically dependent children's program (MDCP) – A Medicaid waiver program that provides nursing, respite and Medicaid benefits to children as an alternative to nursing facility care.

medically necessary care – Care that is provided for the diagnosis or treatment of a condition, judged necessary and appropriate according to the current standards of medical practice, and at an appropriate level of service that can safely be provided. Medically necessary care should be those covered services required to preserve and maintain the health status of a member.

medically needy – Persons who are categorically eligible for Medicaid and whose income, minus total medical bills, is below state income limits for the Medicaid program. *See spend down.*

medically unnecessary days (MUD) – Describes the part of an inpatient stay that is deemed excessive in accordance with the standards of good medical practice. Excessive may be defined as too long a stay or when appropriate care is available in a less costly or more efficient setting.

M

medical management – Techniques used by health insurance and managed care companies to reduce costs and utilization of health care services. An example would be case management. *See case management.*

medical management information system (MMIS) – A data system that allows payers and purchasers to track health care expenditure and utilization patterns.

medical model of health care delivery – Refers to health care that is delivered only when a person is sick, with emphasis placed on diagnosis and treatment of disease rather than health promotion and disease prevention. Health Maintenance Organizations (HMOs) focus on the latter to reduce costs.

medical necessity – A required, indispensable or appropriate procedure; not one provided merely for the convenience of the patient.

medical protocols – *See clinical protocols.*

medical record – A record kept on patients which properly contains sufficient information to identify the patient clearly, to justify his or her diagnosis and treatment, and to document the results accurately.

medical review – Review by a team composed of physicians and other appropriate health and social service personnel of the condition and needs for care, including a medical evaluation, of each inpatient in a long-term care facility.

medical savings account (MSA) – A health care savings account where individuals can accumulate contributions to pay for unreimbursed medical expenses. Individuals could withdraw money only to pay for qualified medical expenses or health insurance premiums. Money in the account not spent can appreciate with interest, and can be used after retirement, somewhat like an IRA. The MSA is used in conjunction with a high-deductible health insurance policy (also called catastrophic coverage), where insurance would pay for expensive treatments that occur infrequently.

MSAs have been around a while, but it wasn't until the Health Insurance Portability and Accountability Act of 1996 that they were more widely recognized. It was this act that allowed the MSA savings to be accumulated on a tax deferred basis. MSAs are most attractive to individuals who anticipate less medical service utilization. MSAs are similar to Flexible Spending Accounts (FSA) which qualify under Section 125 of the IRS Code.

M

Medical Services Organization (MSO) – A health care management entity owned by a hospital, physician organization or third party that provides services such as negotiating fee schedules, managing administrative functions, handling billing and collections, and clinical data management for hospitals and physician groups. *See also management services organization* (MSO).

medical / surgical – Refers to the services performed by a physician. Sometimes abbreviated as med-surg.

Medicare (Title 18) – A nationwide federal health insurance program, created by the 1965 amendment to the Social Security Act, for people aged 65 and over, for persons eligible for Social Security disability payments for over two years, and for certain workers and their dependents who need kidney transplantation or dialysis. Health insurance protection is available to insured persons without regard to income.

Medicare Part A is the hospital insurance program; Part B covers supplementary medical services (physicians' services). Medicare is the secondary payer for disabled beneficiaries under age 65 who have health insurance coverage under a large group plan (100 or more) by reason of their employment or the employment of a family member.

Medicare approved amount – The amount Medicare determines it will pay for a particular service. The individual is responsible for charges above the approved amount unless the doctor or supplier agrees to accept the approved amount as payment in full.

Medicare beneficiary – A patient eligible for Medicare Part B benefits. Patients are usually eligible for Medicare at age 65 and can elect to purchase Part B coverage.

Medicare + Choice (M+C) – Refers to Medicare managed care plans. Congress created the Medicare + Choice program to allow private insurance companies to offer coverage to Medicare beneficiaries. Medicare beneficiaries can choose either the original Medicare plan or a Medicare managed care plan and still receive all services that Medicare covers. Many Medicare managed care plans pay for some extra benefits that the original Medicare plan does not cover, such as limited outpatient prescription drugs or reduced deductibles (what the beneficiary pays before Medicare begins to pay).

Medicare fee schedule – Schedule of Medicare fees based on resource-based relative value scale (RBRVS) factors.

M

Medicare Part A – A federal government program which pays for hospital and institutional type benefits. Specifically, it is the part of Medicare insurance that helps pay for medically necessary inpatient hospital care, and after a hospital stay, for inpatient care in a skilled nursing facility, for home care by a home health agency or hospice care by a licensed and certified hospice agency.

Medicare Part B – A federal government program which pays for physician type benefits. Specifically, it is the part of Medicare insurance that helps pay for medically necessary physician services, outpatient hospital services, outpatient physical therapy, speech pathology services and a number of other medical services and supplies that are not covered by the hospital insurance. Part B will pay for certain inpatient services if the beneficiary does not have Part A.

Medicare Payment Advisory Commission (MedPAC) – A commission mandated by the Balanced Budget Act of 1997 (BBA) to consider, develop, review and advise the U.S. Congress on Medicare policy issues and subsequent improvements. The commission makes policy recommendations based on qualitative and quantitative analyses of relevant issues, discussion of the findings and implications, and deliberations as to the appropriate policy responses. All recommendations are discussed at meetings that are open to the general public.

Medicare risk contract – A contract between a managed care plan and HCFA to provide services to Medicare beneficiaries for a fixed monthly payment. It requires all services be provided by the managed care plan on an at-risk basis. *See Medicare risk HMO.*

Medicare risk HMO – Health plans offered by managed care companies as alternatives to standard Medicare and Medicare supplemental coverage for individuals 65 years of age and older. The premiums are funded by federal health benefits in lieu of Medicare, and members receive care from a specified network of providers who are paid in advance. The plans cover most physician and hospital services, and in some cases, prescriptions and other benefits.

Medicare select – A Medicare supplemental insurance that has lower premiums, but a limited choice of providers. Members may only use providers who have been selected by the insurer as "preferred providers". The exception is emergency care, which can be sought outside the preferred provider network.

Medicare sequence number – HCFA requires that claims submitted by a group practice using a clinic provider number identify the performing physician who rendered each service on the claim form. In

M

order to comply with this requirement, each physician in such a group practice which bills under a clinic provider number has been issued a 4-digit sequence number.

Medicare supplement – Private health insurance plan available to Medicare eligibles to cover the costs of physicians' services and other medical and health services not covered by Medicare. Also called Medigap, Medsupp, or Medicare wrap. Medicare supplement coverage must meet mandatory coverage requirements specified by the federal government.

Medicare wrap – *See Medicare supplement.*

Medigap – *See Medicare supplement.*

MedPAC – *See Medicare Payment Advisory Commission (MedPAC).*

Medsupp – *See Medicare supplement.*

med-surg – An abbreviation for medical / surgical used to refer to managed care organizations that provide acute care benefits. Also pertains to the services performed by a physician.

member – Any person covered under a health plan who is eligible to receive benefits. This term may refer to the subscriber or any of the subscriber's eligible dependents.

member continuity – Continuation of benefits without lapse of coverage when changing from group to group or one health plan program to another.

member month – Used as a unit of volume measurement, a member month is equal to one member enrolled in a managed care plan for one month, whether or not the member actually receives any services during the period. Two member months are equal to one member enrolled for two months or two members enrolled for one month. Many operating figures for managed care companies are expressed in terms of member months (e.g., per member per month (PMPM), per member per year (PMPY), etc.).

membership – The status, including rights, privileges and obligations, of being a subscribing member of a health plan as set forth in its respective bylaws. Membership may include the privilege to apply for enrollment of eligible dependents under a family coverage.

membership agreement – A member's agreement with their health plan, consisting of the written enrollment application of the member and their dependents, including any written health statements required by their health plan and the certificate which includes any

M

authorized amendments issued for attachment.

membership application form – An enrollment form signed by individuals wanting to become members. This form often serves as an agreement between the member and their health plan.

membership benefits – *See benefit, benefit package and benefits.*

membership card – The identification card issued by a health plan as evidence of membership.

membership eligibility tape – Computer tape of required data elements necessary to maintain memberships to pay claims.

membership file – A computer master file of all information pertinent to a member; includes name, certificate number, and contract information.

mental health parity – Refers to efforts by organizations at both the national and state levels to provide equal health insurance coverage for the diagnosis and treatment of mental disorders and substance abuse services as is provided for physical health care.

mental health provider – Psychiatrist, social worker, hospital or other facility licensed to provide mental health services.

mental illness – Any mental disorders listed in the American Psychiatric Association's *Diagnosis and Statistical Manual of Mental Disorders* (DSMIII-R), except mental retardation and learning disabilities. *See Association's Diagnosis and Statistical Manual (DSMIII-R).*

mental retardation – Slowness in intellectual functions that is significantly below the average person.

messenger model – A statement of policy issued jointly by the Federal Trade Commission (FTC) and the Justice Department in 1994 gave the following definition: "A messenger model typically involves an agent or third party conveying to purchasers information obtained individually from providers in the network about the prices the network participants are willing to accept and conveying to providers any contract offers made by purchasers. Each provider then makes an independent, unilateral decision to accept or reject each contract offer."

midlevel practitioner – A term used to describe nurse practitioners (NP), certified nurse-midwives (CNM) and physician assistants (PA) who have been trained to provide medical services that otherwise might be performed by a physician. Midlevel practitioners practice under the supervision of an M.D. or D.O., who takes responsibility

M

for the care they provide. Nurse practitioners (NP) are midlevel practitioners. Also called a midlevel provider, physician extender and non-physician practitioner (NPPs).

midlevel provider – *See midlevel practitioner.*

minimal care – Care rendered to patients who are ambulatory and partially self-sufficient who require limited therapeutic and diagnostic services and are in the final stages of recovery. Focus of nursing management is on maintenance of a therapeutic environment that enhances recovery. Complexity of care includes administering medications and treatments that cannot be done by the patients and providing instruction in self-care and post-hospitalization health maintenance.

minimum premium – Generally, a fully insured funding arrangement which allows the insured to hold the IBNR (incurred but not reported) and reimburse the carrier for paid claims as they emerge. Minimum premium arrangements were originally developed by commercial carriers to minimize state premium taxes.

miscellaneous expenses – Expenses in connection with hospital insurance; for example, hospital charges other than room and board, such as x-rays, drugs, laboratory fees and other ancillary charges.

mission statement – A general statement that describes a company's reason for existence, its vision and direction, its areas of expertise and its goals.

MMIS – *See medical management information system.*

modality – The methods of treatment, including the conditions under which symptoms develop and become better or worse.

Modified Community Rating (MCR) – A community rating impacted by health care usage in a given geographic area using such factors as age, sex, etc. Compare to adjusted community rating (ACR).

modified fee-for-service – A system that pays providers fees for services provided, with a set maximum fee for each service. *See also fee-for-service* (FFS).

monthly increment process – The process of applying one or two months' dues when receivables have been created for quarterly or annual dues.

moral hazard – Refers to the phenomenon that patients are more likely to abuse a service if they believe that someone else is paying for it. Health care has a high moral hazard component because there

M

is no incentive built into the system to encourage the reduction of costs.

morbidity – The incidence of disease, injury or disability in a defined population, usually expressed in general or specific rates of incidence or prevalence. *See incidence and prevalence.*

morbidity rate – An actuarial term showing likelihood of medical expenses occurring. *See actuarial.*

morbidity table – The incidence and severity of sicknesses and accidents in a well-defined class or classes of persons. It is used to forecast the rate of occurrence of disability. *See actuarial.*

mortality – Death. The term "mortality" is used to describe the relation of deaths to the population in which they occur. *See mortality rate.*

mortality rate – Expresses the number of deaths in a unit of population within a prescribed time or for specific diseases. Mortality rates are also used to state death rates for such variables as age, sex, or other demographic variables.

mortality table – Used to forecast the rate of death, usually on the basis of tracing the year by year history of a group of individuals from birth until death.

MRI – Magnetic Resonance Imaging. A diagnostic testing process using an electron magnet that produces a computer enhanced magnetic field that produces a "picture" similar to an x-ray or CT scan (computed tomography). Both x-rays and CT scans make radiograph images (photographic negatives).

MSA – *See medical savings account.*

MSO – *See medical services organization or management services organization.*

multiple employer trust (MET) – A group of small, unrelated employers who join together for the purpose of providing group medical coverage on an insured or self-funded basis. By banding together, a multiple employer trust broadens the membership pool, preventing adverse selection and resulting in lower health insurance costs. METs are similar to health plan purchasing cooperatives (HPPC), but smaller in scale. *See health plan purchasing cooperatives* (HPPC).

multiple employer welfare arrangement (MEWA) – As defined in ERISA (Employee Retirement Income Security Act), an employee welfare benefit plan or any other arrangement providing benefits to the employees of two or more employers. *See multiple employer trust* (MET).

M

multiple option plan – A plan where employees are offered a choice of health plans from their employer; for instance, a Heath Maintenance Organization (HMO), preferred provider organization (PPO) or indemnity plan. Employers establish the contribution they will make toward the health premiums, with the rest being paid for by the employee, usually through payroll deductions. Plans that have "richer benefits" (e.g., HMO or POS) typically cost employees less than those plans that allow more "freedom of choice" (PPO or indemnity). *See Health Maintenance Organization* (HMO), *preferred provider organization* (PPO), *and point of service* (POS).

multiple surgical procedure – Two or more surgeries performed on a patient during the same operative session.

multi-specialty group – Refers to physicians from various primary and specialty practices that work together in a group practice.

NAIC – *See National Association of Insurance Commissioners.*

National Association of Blue Shield Plans (NABSP) – Former name of the national coordinating organization for all Blue Shield plans, now merged and called Blue Cross and Blue Shield Association (BCBSA).

National Association of Insurance Commissioners (NAIC) – A national association of insurance commissioners from various states formed to promote national uniformity in the regulation of insurance.

National Committee on Quality Assurance (NCQA) – A non-profit organization created to improve patient care quality and health plan performance in partnership with managed care plans, purchasers, consumers, and the public sector. NCQA reviews managed care organizations in the areas of quality management, utilization management, physician credentialing, members' rights and responsibilities, preventive health services, and medical records and accredits those plans that meet their standards. NCQA awards the following types of status:

- *Applied*—The managed care plan has applied to NCQA for review.
- *Denied*—The plan does not qualify for any of the other NCQA accreditation categories.
- *Full*—The plan has excellent quality improvement programs, meets rigorous standards and is accredited for three years.
- *None*—The plan has not applied for NCQA accreditation.
- *One year*—The plan has well-established quality improvement programs, meets most NCQA standards, and will be reviewed again in a year to determine if it can move up to full accreditation.
- *Pending*—The plan has been reviewed by NCQA and accreditation status is pending.
- *Provisional*—Granted for one year to plans that have adequate quality improvement programs and meet some NCQA standards, but need to demonstrate progress before they can qualify for higher levels of accreditation.
- *Scheduled*—The plan has scheduled an NCQA review.
- *Under Review*—NCQA has given the plan an accreditation status, which is being reconsidered at the request of the plan.

National Drug Code (NDC) – A national classification system for the identification of drugs, similar to the universal product code (UPC) used for manufactured goods.

N

national health expenditures (NHE) – An economic indicator to show what the U.S. spends on health care annually, expressed as a percentage of the gross domestic product (GDP). The NHE is the sum total of all health care expenditures, including physician and hospital services, drugs, home nursing care, dental services, administrative costs, research, etc.

national health insurance – A proposal to make government the single payer for all health care. National health insurance is a highly debated subject among politicians, providers and businesses. The pro-national health insurance supporters state that, If implemented, it would provide "universal coverage" for all citizens, similar to health plans in Great Britain and Canada. Anti-national health insurance forces contend that if the government administers the program, businesses will have to fund it. *See universal coverage.*

national practitioner data bank (NPDB) – A central repository of information on physicians, dentists, and in some cases, other health care practitioners that began operations on September 1, 1990. It contains reports on medical malpractice payments, adverse licensure actions, adverse clinical privilege actions, and adverse professional society membership actions. Information that is reported to the NPDB is available to hospitals, other health care entities that provide health care services and have a formal review process, professional societies, state licensing boards, plaintiff's attorneys and pro se plaintiffs (those representing themselves) under limited circumstances, researchers (statistical data only), and health care practitioners (self-query only). Hospitals are required to request reports from the NPDB when a physician or dentist applies for staff privileges. Related to the healthcare integrity and protection data bank (HIPDB). Both the NPDB and HIPDB are administered by a division of the Health Resources and Services Administration (HRSA) within the U.S. Department of Health and Human Services (HHS).

naturopathy – The system of medicine where only natural medicines and methods are used, including fresh food, exercise, massage, hygiene, light, etc.

NCQA – *See National Committee on Quality Assurance.*

NDC – *See National Drug Code.*

needs assessment – Evaluation of the requirements or demands for health services by a population or community.

Neo ICU – *See neonatal intensive care unit.*

N

neonatal intensive care unit (Neo ICU or NICU) – A hospital unit with special equipment for the care of premature and seriously ill newborn infants.

neonatology – The study of the treatment and care of premature and/or high-risk newborn babies.

nephrology – Diagnosis and non-surgical treatment of diseases and disorders of the kidney, including kidney dialysis.

net loss ratio – Total claims liability and total expenses divided by premiums.

network – A group of doctors, hospitals, pharmacies and other health care providers who, through formal and informal contracts, provide health care services to members of a health plan. Networks may contract externally to obtain administrative and financial services.

network model HMO – A Health Maintenance Organization (HMO) that contracts with two or more independent group practices (single and multi-specialty groups) to provide health care to its members. The physicians work out of their own office, but do not necessarily provide care exclusively for HMO members. For federal qualification purposes, network models are designated as individual practice associations (IPAs). Compare to a direct contracting, group model HMO, and individual practice association (IPA).

neurology – Medical diagnosis and treatment of disorders of the nervous system.

neurosurgery – Diagnosis and surgery of the nervous system and brain.

new cost funding – A conventionally insured, experienced-rated contract that refunds any cash surpluses to members while limiting the amount that they may carryover to the next year.

NF – Nursing facility.

NICU – *See neonatal intensive care unit.*

non-contributory – A term applied to employee benefit plans under which the employer bears the full cost of the benefits for the employees. One hundred percent of the eligible employees must be insured.

non-duplication of benefits – This is a particular exclusion in some health care coverage contracts. It is different than coordination of benefits in that any services covered in whole or part by another

N

program are excluded from coverage.

non-group – A pool of subscribers having no affiliation with a company-sponsored group. A non-group is enrolled direct.

non-member hospital – A hospital which has not entered into an agreement with a health insurance plan to provide hospital services to its members.

non-par – Abbreviation for non-participating provider (physician or hospital).

non-participating hospital – *See non-member hospital.*

non-participating provider (non-par) – A provider who has not entered into an agreement with a health insurance plan to provide medical services to its members and, therefore, expects to be paid the full amount of the fees charged for services performed.

nonphysician practitioners (NPPs) – *See midlevel practitioner.*

non-plan provider – A health care provider without a contract with an insurer.

non-residential treatment center – A facility which can provide medical and other services for the treatment of alcoholism, substance abuse, and/or psychiatric problems to individuals who do not require inpatient status and are free from acute physical and mental complications. The facility must maintain an organized program of treatment which may be limited to less than 12 hours per day and not be available seven days a week. Facility must be accredited by JCAHO and be certified or licensed as such by the state of Missouri.

non-systemic condition – A condition that is localized and affects one particular area of the body (e.g., kidney stones, ear disorders, cataracts, bunions, torn knee cartilage, etc.).

nosocomial – Pertaining to or originating in a hospital.

notice of admission – This form is sent to a health insurance plan by the hospital when a member is admitted for inpatient care. The form contains the patient's name, address, sex, age, admission date, certificate number and the reason for admission.

NPDB – *See National Practitioner Data Bank.*

nurse – Person qualified by graduation from a formal nursing program at an accredited school of nursing and licensed by a state to practice nursing.

N

nurse midwife, certified (CNM) – *See certified nurse-midwife* (CNM).

nurse practitioner (NP) – A registered nurse (RN) with advanced academic and clinical training that provides care similar to a physician, but with limited scope. Nurse practitioners function under the supervision of a physician and emphasize preventive medicine. Their services include the diagnosis and treatment of acute and chronic diseases, counseling patients, and prescribing medications. They are often utilized in physician offices to handle routine patient cases or conditions, freeing up physicians for more difficult ones. NPs have been successfully employed in a variety of specialties, particularly pediatrics, neonatology, women's health and geriatrics. Many nurse practitioners are certified in their specialty field. NPs are considered mid-level providers.

nurse triage – Nurses screen telephone calls from patients to provide faster access and appropriate care by using a technique in which patients are "sorted" by the type of injury or disorder and its severity on the basis of medically approved guidelines. Managed care organizations use triage to direct care and efficiently use resources, as well as for utilization review. Also called telephone triage system. *See triage and referral center.*

nursing – Provision of services, by or under the direction of a nurse, to patients requiring assistance in recovering or maintaining their physical or mental health.

nursing home – A wide range of institutions, other than hospitals, which provide various levels of maintenance, personal care or nursing care to people who are unable to care for themselves. Nursing home residents have diverse health problems ranging from minimal to very serious.

nursing facility – A facility licensed by and approved by each state in which eligible individuals receive nursing care and appropriate rehabilitative and restorative services under the Title XIX (Medicaid) long-term care program.

nursing notes – Detailed records of care rendered to a patient which are prepared by the attending nurse and become part of the patient's medical records.

OA – *See open access.*

OBRA – *See Omnibus Budget Reconciliation Act (OBRA).*

observation unit – A particular area in the hospital for the purpose of observing patients' disorders and/or complications for no longer than 23 hours and 59 minutes. This is the typical standard at which time the patient is usually released or admitted and transferred to an inpatient unit. The majority of observation unit patients come from the emergency room.

obsolete care – Care that, in the judgment of the health insurance company, is no longer generally accepted as standard care according to the prevalent standards of medical care practice.

obstetrical services – Medical care and/or surgery rendered by a physician (usually an obstetrician) or other licensed health care professional in connection with pregnancy or delivery (childbirth), including the usual prenatal and postnatal care.

obstetrics (OB) – The specialty of medicine that is concentrated on the care of women during pregnancy and childbirth.

occupancy rate – A measure of inpatient health facility use determined by dividing the number of available bed days by patient days. Occupancy rate measures the average percentage of a hospital's beds occupied and may be institution-wide or specific for one department or service.

occupational therapist – An individual qualified by graduation from an accredited school of occupational therapy with either a baccalaureate or masters degree who has passed a national certification examination given by the American Occupational Therapy Association. In many states, a license to practice is also required. *See occupational therapy services.*

occupational therapy services – Department which provides occupational therapy interventions in a medical community setting by evaluating patients' performance capabilities and deficits, and planning and implementing occupational therapy services in prevention, health maintenance, remediation, daily life tasks and vocational adjustments health care programs.

OCL – *See other carrier liability.*

Office of Health Maintenance Organizations – The office of the U.S.

O

Department of Health and Human Services (HHS) responsible for directing the federal HMO program.

OHMO – *See Office of Health Maintenance Organizations.*

ombudsperson – A person within a managed care organization or outside of the health care system who is designated to receive and investigate complaints about quality of care, inability to access care, discrimination and other problems that beneficiaries may experience with their managed care organization. The ombudsperson acts as the beneficiary's advocate in pursuing grievances or complaints.

Omnibus Budget Reconciliation Act (OBRA) – Federal laws that direct how federal monies are to be expended. Amendments to Medicare and Medicaid eligibility and benefit rules, as well as reimbursements, are frequently made in such acts.

OOA – *See out-of-area.*

OOPs – *See out-of-pocket expense.*

OP – Abbreviation for outpatient. *See outpatient.*

OPD – *See outpatient diagnostic rider.*

open access – A term that describes a member's ability to self-refer for specialty care. In open access plans members are allowed to receive services outside the provider network without referral authorization, but are usually required to pay an additional co-pay and/or deductible. Typically found in an individual practice association (IPA) and a Health Maintenance Organization (HMO). Also called open panel or open-ended.

open-ended – *See open access.*

open enrollment (open enrollment period) – A time period, often once a year, when new subscribers may elect to enroll in, or transfer between, health insurance plans offered by their employer. During this time, Health Maintenance Organizations (HMOs) must accept all applicants of a group without evidence of insurability or waiting periods. Federal HMO regulations require HMOs that meet certain criteria to conduct annual open enrollments for periods of not less than 30 days.

open formulary – A listing of drugs a health plan prefers, but does not require physicians to prescribe for their patients who are health plan members.

O

open panel – Private physicians willing to accept a health plan's terms to provide care in their own offices. *See open access.*

operating bed – A bed that is currently set up and ready in all respects for the care of a patient. It must include supporting space, equipment and staff to operate under normal circumstances. Excluded are transient patient beds, bassinets, incubators, labor beds and recovery beds.

operative notes – The detail records prepared by the operating surgeon(s) pertaining to a patient's surgical procedure. Operative notes are part of the patient's medical records.

ophthalmologist – A person licensed to practice ophthalmology, the branch of medicine that deals with the diagnosis and treatment of disorders and diseases of the eye.

ophthalmology – Medical and surgical treatment of diseases and disorders of the eye, including the evaluation of vision and prescription of lenses for visual problems.

ophthalmologist – A physician who specializes in ophthalmology, the branch of medicine that deals with the diagnosis and treatment of disorders and diseases of the eye.

OPL – *See other party liability.*

OPM – Office of personnel management. This is the U.S. Government entity that controls the Federal Employee Health Benefits Program.

optician – Any individual or company that makes or dispenses eyeglasses prescribed by ophthalmologists or optometrists to correct visual defects in the eye. Specifically, the optician grinds the lenses or has them ground according to prescription, fits them into a frame and adjusts the frame to fit the face.

optional benefits – Benefits that may be purchased along with the standard programs. For example, benefits for mental illness treatment or chemical dependency and drug addiction treatment. *For Medicaid definition, see optional services or benefits.*

optional services or benefits – Over 30 different services which a state can elect to cover under a state Medicaid plan, as defined by the Health Care Financing Administration (HCFA). Examples include personal care, rehabilitative services, prescription drugs, therapies, diagnostic services, ICF-MR, and targeted case management.

optometrist – A person licensed to practice optometry (the measurement/correction and fitting of lenses).

O

organized care system – An advanced form of an integrated delivery system (IDS) resulting from mergers, linkages and affiliations between physicians, health systems and managed care organizations. *See integrated delivery system.*

orthopedics (orthopaedics) – Surgical and medical treatment of ligaments, joints, muscles, tendons and related structures.

osteopathy – A system of medicine which emphasizes the theory that the body can make its own remedies, given normal structural relationships, environmental conditions, and nutrition. It differs from allopathy primarily in its greater attention to body mechanics and manipulative methods in diagnosis and therapy. Osteopathy is second to allopathy in number of practitioners in the United States. Osteopathic physicians are granted the Doctor of Osteopathy (DO). *See Doctor of Osteopathy* (DO).

OTC – *See over-the-counter drug.*

other carrier liability (OCL) – A term used in the coordination of benefits (COB) describing the decision that the other plan is the primary plan. OCL is also used for workers compensation and carve-out programs to describe when another party is the primary payer. Sometimes called other party liability (OPL).

other medical expenses (OME) – Generally, those medical expenses excluding institutional charges.

other party liability (OPL) – *See other carrier liability* (OCL).

otolaryngologist – A physician with specialty in the medical and surgical treatment of the head and neck, including ears, nose and throat. Also called ENT, for ear, nose and throat.

otolaryngology – Medical and surgical treatment of the head and neck, including ears, nose and throat.

outcome indicators – Certain outcomes of care that can be identified and are subject to analysis (e.g., neonatal death rate, mortality following coronary artery bypass surgery, readmission rate following discharge and nosocomial infection rate).

outcomes – Results that are achieved through a given health care service, preventive health measure, prescription drug use, or medical procedure. Essentially, the results of patient care. Managed care organizations are developing comprehensive systems for measuring and improving outcomes.

outcomes management – Refers to systematically improving health

O

care results by utilizing data gleaned from outcomes measurement. By utilizing a database of outcomes experience, providers will know which treatment modalities result in consistently better outcomes for patients. Specifically, outcomes management means re-measuring outcomes and re-modifying treatment modalities continuously, possibly with the intention of developing clinical protocols or practice guidelines.

outcomes measurement – The formal process of systematically measuring individual or collective clinical treatment, and response to that treatment (outcomes).

outcomes measures – Assessments which gauge the effect or results of treatment for a particular disease or condition. Outcome measures include, but are not limited to, objective of mortality, morbidity and health status, as well as subjective data such as the patient's perception of restoration of function, quality of life and functional status.

outcomes research – Studies aimed at measuring the effect of specific medical and health interventions on health or health care costs. The difficulty in outcomes research is differentiating between the results of health care treatments and the substantial amount of other factors that may also affect patients' health and satisfaction.

outlier – A patient whose length of stay (LOS) or treatment cost differs substantially from the normal length of stays or costs of other patients in a diagnosis related group (DRG). The term is most often used in utilization review. Also called day outlier or stay outlier.

outlier thresholds – The day and cost cut-off points that separate inlier patients from outlier patients.

out-of-area (OOA) – Health care obtained by a covered person outside the network service area.

out-of-area benefits – The coverage allowed to HMO members for services outside of the prescribed geographic area of the HMO. These benefits usually include emergency care and provisions for out-of-state students. Some HMOs offer low fee-for-service payments for non-emergency care. Members may need to file claim forms for reimbursement of their out-of-pocket expenses for these benefits.

out-of-area services – *See out-of-area benefits.*

out-of-hospital psychiatric care – Mental health care provided in the physician's office and predominantly involving psychoanalysis.

O

out-of-network – Providers who do not participate in the network of a managed care plan. Members of managed care plans are encouraged to avoid using physicians who are out-of-network. HMO members usually have to pay for out-of-network services themselves, while POS members might be covered, but at a reduced benefit level compared to in-network providers.

out-of-network benefits – Refers to the reimbursement a member will receive from a health plan for services provided by a hospital or doctor that is "out-of-network." Some preferred provider organizations (PPOs) have provisions for using "out-of-network" providers, usually in conjunction with a higher copay or a lower reimbursement. With most HMOs, a patient is not reimbursed for services delivered by out-of-network providers. *See out-of-network.*

out-of-pocket expense (OOPs) – Any medical care costs not covered by insurance, which must be paid by the insured. Out-of-pocket expenses include copayments, coinsurance and deductibles. Sometimes called direct costs.

out-of-pocket limit – *See out-of-pocket maximum.*

out-of-pocket maximum – The maximum amount an employee has to pay in any year toward the cost of medical treatment; usually the total of the deductible and coinsurance amounts.

out-of-pocket payments – *See out-of-pocket expense.*

outpatient (OP) – A participant who receives health care provided by a hospital or other qualified facility, but does not occupy a bed. Some health care plans define outpatient as a person who receives health care and is discharged within 23 hours (more hours would define the person as an inpatient).

outpatient diagnostic rider (OPD) – Benefits that can be added to a health plan to provide coverage for diagnostic studies and tests for the diagnosis and treatment of illness or injury in the outpatient department of a hospital.

out-patient facility – Health care facilities that provide outpatient care. Facilities include hospitals, mental health clinics, rural health clinics, mobile x-ray units, or free-standing dialysis units.

outpatient hospital claim – A request for benefit payments for outpatient services.

outpatient review – A review of outpatient services that assures the appropriateness of treatment and monitors ongoing care.

O

outpatient services – Medical and other services provided by a hospital or other qualified facility to a patient on an outpatient basis. Services can include surgical procedures, rehabilitation therapy, physical therapy, occupational therapy, diagnostic x-ray and laboratory tests. *See outpatient.*

outpatient surgery – Surgical procedures performed on patients who are not admitted to a hospital.

outpatient visit – *See ambulatory visit.*

overcoding – *See upcoding.*

over-the-counter drug (OTC) – A drug that does not require a prescription under federal or state law, and therefore may be advertised and sold directly to the public without a prescription.

overage – Credit to group or subscriber's billing.

override – A claims adjudication action taken when the computerized (automated) logic is not used to finalize a claim. Instead, the adjudicator tells the computer what to pay to whom. In other words, the adjudicator overrides the system.

PAC – Pre-admission certification. *See pre-certification.*

package – A combination of contracts where each contract identifies a particular type of benefit; for example, dental, behavioral health, etc. There may be several packages within one group.

packaged pricing – *See global pricing.*

paid as billed – Dues paid exactly as billed with no subscriber maintenance or changes.

paid claim – A claim that has been charged to the experience of a program once a check has either been issued to the payee, or, alternatively, has been issued and has cleared the banking system.

paid claims loss ratio – *See loss ratio.*

P&T – *See pharmacy and therapeutics committee (P&T).*

panel – Private physicians willing to accept the plan's terms to provide care in their own offices.

PAR – Abbreviation for participating provider (physician or hospital). *See participating provider.*

partial disability – When a person can perform some, but not all of the duties of their occupation. Also refers to when the patient has permanently lost a specific percentage of his or her earning capacity.

partial hospitalization – Formal programs of care in a hospital or other institution for periods of less than 24 hours a day, typically involving services usually provided to inpatients.

partially self-funded – *See self-insurance or self-insured.*

participant – *See member.*

participating dentist – A dentist who has entered into an agreement with a health insurance plan to provide dental services to its members.

participating hospital – A hospital that has entered into an agreement with a health insurance plan to provide hospital services to its members.

participating pharmacy – A pharmacy that has entered into an agreement with a health insurance plan to provide medical services to its members.

P

participating physician – A physician who has entered into an agreement with a health insurance plan to provide medical services to its members.

participating provider (PAR) – A provider who has entered into an agreement with a health insurance plan to provide medical services to its members. The provider may be a hospital, pharmacy or other facility or a physician who has contractually accepted the terms and conditions as set forth by the health plan. Also called affiliated health care provider.

pass through – *See first pass.*

pathology – Laboratory study of body tissue and fluids to diagnose disease.

patient – A person who is receiving health services.

patient acuity – Measures the intensity of care required for a patient based on six categories ranging from minimal care (I) to intensive care (VI).

patient liability – The dollar amount that a patient is legally obligated to pay for services that are provided by a hospital, physician or clinician.

patient mix – The numbers and types of patients served by a hospital or other health program. Patients may be classified according to their homes, socioeconomic characteristics, diagnosis, or severity of illness.

patient origin study – A study to determine the geographic distribution of patients served by one or more health programs. These studies are usually conducted by hospital systems, health plans or health planning agencies to determine the effectiveness of current health programs and to define catchment areas and medical trade areas. Patient origin studies are also highly useful in the planning and development of new health care services. *See catchment area.*

patient panel – The population of patients (members) assigned to a provider by a health care plan.

pay or play – A health care proposal that would require all employers to either provide medical insurance for their workers or pay a tax that would enable government to provide it.

pay and pursue – A term used to explain that coordination of benefits (COB) provisions are administered after payment of a claim. Hence, the claim is paid and then COB is pursued.

P

payer – Any individual or organizations that purchases health care services. Sometimes called payor.

payor – *See payer.*

PBM – *See pharmacy benefit manager.*

PCCM – *See primary care case management.*

PCN – *See primary care network.*

PCP – *See primary care physician.*

PCP capitation – *See capitation.*

PCPM – Per contract per month. *See per member per month.*

PCR – Physician contingency reserve. *See withhold.*

PDR – *Physician's Desk Reference* (PDR).

PEC – *See pre-existing condition* (PEC).

pediatrician – A physician that specializes in the study and treatment of disease and disorders of children.

pediatrics – The study and treatment of disease and disorders of children.

pediatric oncology – Diagnosis and treatment of diseases and disorders of the blood, cancer, hematology/ and tumors in children.

peer review – Confidential processes in which physicians review each other's practice activities for appropriateness and quality of patient care. A review may also include clinical performance of all individuals with delineated clinical privileges. For specific cases, peer review providers receive copies of the patient's chart and other relevant clinical information, review the case, and then discuss it with the treating provider.

Peer Review Organization (PRO) – An organization established by TEFRA (Tax Equity and Fiscal Responsibility Act of 1982) to review quality of care and appropriateness of admissions, readmissions and discharges for Medicare and Medicaid. The physician-sponsored and operated organization is responsible for reviewing health care services provided to patients to determine their appropriateness, necessity, quality and reasonableness. As such, the duties of PROs include arbitrating disagreements between or among doctors, dentists, patients or third parties. PROs replace Professional Standards Review Organizations (PSROs).

P

penetration – The percentage of business that a health plan is able to capture of a particular population or in the market area as a whole. For example, an HMO that signs up 40,000 members out of 400,000 in a market has 10% market penetration.

per case payment – A method used primarily to pay providers on a prospective basis. In most cases, the payment is made by type of case without regard to services rendered.

per contract per month (PCPM) – *See per member per month* (PMPM).

per diem cost – Cost per day for hospital or other institutional care including all supplies and services provided to the patient during the day, but excluding the professional fees of non-staff physicians.

per diem payment – A rate of payment on a daily basis.

per diem rate – Contracted amounts paid for inpatient stays, calculated per day per type of stay.

performance goals – *See performance standards.*

performance standards – The standards an individual provider is expected to meet, especially with respect to quality of care. Performance standards are usually set up in group practices and may include office hours per week, office visits per month, on-call days, collections as a percentage of charges, operations performed per year, etc.

periodic interim payment (PIP) – The prepayment of benefits to a provider based on historic utilization of that provider by members. This is a cash flow leveling benefit to providers.

permanent disability –
  1. A disability from which the insured individual does not recover.
  2. An injured employee's diminished capacity to return to work. The employee is not expected to be able to return to the job they held before the illness or injury, or to have any other form of employment.

per member per month (PMPM) – Refers to the cost or revenue from each plan's member for one month; the unit of measure related to each effective member for each month the member was effective. The calculation is the number of units/member months (MM). PMPM specifically applies to a revenue or cost for each enrolled member each month. Variations include PSPM (per subscriber per month) and PCPM (per contract per month).

P

per member per year (PMPY) – Same as per member per month, but calculations are based on a year.

per thousand members per year (PTMPY) – A common way of reporting utilization for health plan members. An example would be hospital utilization expressed as days PTMPY.

personal care – Optional Medicaid benefit which allows a state to provide attendant services to assist functionally impaired individuals in performing the Activities of Daily Living (ADL), including bathing, dressing, feeding and grooming. *See Activities of Daily Living.*

phantom providers – Practitioners from whom the patient does not receive direct services separately, but for which they get billed. Examples include anesthesiologists, radiologists and pathologists.

pharmacoeconomics – The study of the cost effectiveness of interventions such as drugs or surgical procedures on patient care.

pharmacy – Any establishment which is registered as a pharmacy with the appropriate state licensing agency and in which prescription drugs are regularly compounded and dispensed by a licensed pharmacist.

pharmacy and therapeutics committee (P&T) – A panel of physicians from multi-specialties who advise the health care plan on the safe and effective use of prescription medications. One major responsibility of the panel is to develop, manage and administer a drug formulary.

pharmacy benefit manager – A health care provider organization that specializes in managing the drug benefit for health plans or employers using managed care principles. Also called a pharmacy benefit management organization.

pharmacy benefit management organization – *See pharmacy benefit manager.*

pharmacy claims – A bill generated for payment as a result of a members' use of prescription drugs dispensed by a pharmacist under a physician's instructions.

pharmacy network – *See pharmacy services administrative organization (PSAO).*

pharmacy services administrative organization (PSAO) – Also known as a pharmacy network, a PSAO is a preferred provider organization (PPO) of community pharmacies. The network contracts either with employers or to pharmacy benefit managers (PBMs) to provide

P

pharmacy services to their enrollees. *See pharmacy benefit manager* (PBM).

PHARMD – Doctor of Pharmacy. *See pharmacy.*

PHO – *See physician/hospital organization.*

PHP – *See prepaid health plan.*

physical therapist – An individual qualified by graduation from an accredited school of physical therapy with either a baccalaureate or masters degree and licensed by a state licensing board to practice physical therapy.

physical therapy services – Activities related to the evaluation of patients with neuromusculoskeletal complaints, and the planning of programs for the physical rehabilitation of patients who may have been referred by either physicians or dentists.

physician – A duly licensed Doctor of Medicine (M.D.) or Doctor of Osteopathy (D.O.) who is not an intern, a resident or in training.

physician agreement – The legal agreement between a managed care company and a participating physician.

physician assistant (PA) – A health care professional who provides basic health care services to patients under the supervision of a physician. PAs are qualified to take medical histories, perform physical examinations, order and interpret lab tests, diagnose and treat conditions, assist in surgery, prescribe and dispense medication and counsel patients.

To qualify as a PA, individuals must successfully complete an intensive PA education program accredited by the Commission on Accreditation of Allied Health Education Programs. Following graduation, they take a national certification exam developed by the National Commission on Certification of PAs, in conjunction with the National Board of Medical Examiners. States require graduation from an accredited PA program and passage of the national certifying exam for licensure. To maintain their national certification, PAs must log 100 hours of continuing medical education (CME) every two years, and sit for a recertification every six years. Also known as a physician extender, mid-level practitioner or mid-level provider.

physician attestation – The requirement that the attending physician certify, in writing, the accuracy and completion of the clinical information used for DRG assignment.

P

physician contingency reserve (PCR) – See *withhold*.

physician Current Procedural Terminology (CPT) – See *Current Procedural Terminology* (CPT).

physician extender (PE) – Health care professionals that help to "extend" health practices by substituting for physicians in performing basic medical services. For example, counseling patients, taking medical histories, seeing acute care patients, etc. A physician assistant is a physician extender. See *midlevel practitioner*.

physician hospital organization (PHO) – An organizational entity that is formed between hospitals and physicians primarily to pursue managed care contracts. The organizational structure furthers cooperative activity while allowing a level of independence to the participating parties. The PHO serves as a negotiating, contracting and marketing unit, and offers health plan enrollees a "seamless" continuum of care. It can also provide management services and other services typically associated with an MSO. The PHO is often superseded by a medical foundation, which is more integrated in its governance and operation. See *integrated delivery system, management services organization, medical services organization, and medical foundation*.

physician incentive plan (PIP) – Refers to any physician compensation plan based on the use or cost of referral services. Physician incentive plan is designated in the Health Care Financing Administration (HCFA) rules that apply to Medicare risk contracts, Medicaid Health Maintenance Organizations (HMOs) and health insuring organizations contracting under Medicare that are subject to the Social Security Act.

Under these rules, managed care organizations (MCOs) need to report the details on PIPs between groups and individual physicians if those physicians are placed at substantial financial risk (SFR); that is, if the compensation plan is based on the use or cost of referral services. Incentive plans may not be based on the refusal or denial of service to Medicare and Medicaid beneficiaries.

physician licensing boards – Organizations that exist in each state with responsibility for issuing the license, accreditation, or certification necessary for a health care provider to practice in the state. These organizations can answer any questions about laws regarding licensing of physicians or whether a particular physician is licensed in that state. Physician licensing boards are also called medical licensing board, Board of Medical Practice, Department of Business and Professional Regulation, Board of Healing Arts and Board of Medical Examiners.

P

physician organization (PO) – An organized group of physicians who come together to contract with managed care companies as one entity or to represent the physician component in a physician hospital organization (PHO). The PO links information systems and integrates practice financials to allow the physicians to manage risk and capitation.

physician payment review commission (PPRC) – A bipartisan congressional advisory group established in 1986 to recommend changes in current reimbursement procedures and policies for physicians receiving payments from Medicare and Medicaid. The commission prepares an annual report to Congress, and in 1990, its responsibilities were expanded to include other payment policy issues.

***Physicians' Desk Reference* (PDR)** – An annual compendium of information concerning prescription drugs and diagnostic products published primarily for physicians and widely used as a reference document.

***Physicians' Office Manual* (POM)** – An informative manual prepared and periodically updated by the provider relations departments of managed care companies. It serves as a useful instructional and reference source for medical assistants in a physicians office, providing claim filing instructions, a guide for obtaining telephone assistance, samples of account ID cards, etc.

physician practice management company (PPMC) – An investor-owned business that purchases, partners with or manages physician practices. The PPMC provides investment capital for a practice's development or expansion.

physician profiling – *See profiling.*

physician visits – Refers to health plan coverage that provides reimbursement for physician's fees for visits in cases of injury or sickness. Health plan coverage can be for either in-hospital visits only or for in-hospital visits and doctor visits out of the hospital setting.

PIP – *See periodic interim payment.*

plan administration – The management unit responsible for running and controlling a managed care plan. Plan administration includes such functions as accounting, billing, underwriting, servicing of accounts, marketing, and legal.

plan age – The number of years that a health plan has been in operation. Usually applied to HMOs.

P

plan area – The area served by the health care plan.

plan document – The document that contains all of the provisions, conditions and terms of operation of a health plan (claims filing, payment of claims, deductibles, prescription drug plan, coordination of benefits, administrative rules, etc.). A plan document may be written in technical terms in contrast to a summary plan description (SPD) which, under the Employee Retirement Income Security Act (ERISA), must be written in language simple enough to be understood by the average plan participant. Also called a health plan document.

plan year – The benefit year that the plan is in effect.

planning approval – The approval of a new health care facility, addition or new equipment through the mechanism established pursuant to any federal or state law. *See certificate of need* (CON).

play or pay – System in which employers must either provide health insurance for their employees or pay a tax to offset governmental costs incurred by providing coverage.

PMPM – *See per member per month.*

PMPY – *See per member per year.*

PO – *See physician organization.*

podiatrist – *See Doctor of Podiatric Medicine* (DPM).

podiatry – The study of the diagnosis and treatment of disorders of the foot and ankle. Sometimes called chiropody, although this is considered an obsolete term.

point-of-care technology – Technologies that enable physicians and other clinicians to electronically record findings, enter orders, and review information from the location where care is provided. Point-of-care technology is at the heart of telemedicine. *See telemedicine.*

point of service (POS) – A form of managed care that combines the rich benefits and low costs of an HMO plan (in-network) with the higher costs, but greater freedom of a PPO plan (out-of-network). This health care delivery system is sometimes called an open-ended HMO or PPO. Members are encouraged to choose a primary care physician and utilize the existing network providers, but have free choice of physicians and hospitals for many services.

When a member uses a participating provider, benefits are provided as an HMO (no deductibles, coinsurance, and small co-pays). If

P

the provider is not part of the designated provider network, members are required to pay a higher co-payment and often a substantial deductible. POSs are fast becoming one of the most popular plans, and represent the area of greatest HMO growth.

policy – The legal documents issued by the company to the policyholder that outlines the conditions and terms of the insurance. Also called the policy contract and the contract. *See contract.*

policy contract – *See policy and contract.*

POM – *See Physician's Office Manual.*

pool – *See risk pool.*

pooling – Combining risks for groups into one risk pool. *See risk.*

population-based care – *See disease management.*

population-based care management – *See disease management.*

population per HMO – The ratio of a metropolitan area market population divided by the number of HMOs operating in that market area. For example, a market population of 1 million people divided by 10 HMOs in the market equals 100,000 population per HMO.

portability – Provides access to continuous health coverage so the insured does not lose insurance coverage due to any change in health or personal status (such as employment, marriage or divorce). *See Health Insurance Portability and Accountability Act of 1996 (HIPAA).*

power of attorney – Authority given one person or corporation to act for and obligate another, to the extent laid down in the instrument creating the power.

PPMC – *See physician practice management company.*

PPO – *See preferred provider organization.*

PPRC – *See Physician Payment Review Commission.*

PPS – *See prospective payment system.*

practical nurses – Practical nurses, also known as vocational nurses, provide nursing care and treatment of patients under the supervision of a licensed physician or registered nurse (RN). Licensure as either a licensed practical nurse (LPN) or, in California and Texas, as a licensed vocational nurse (LVN), is required.

practice guidelines – Defined by the American Medical Association as

P

strategies for patient management, developed to assist physicians in making decisions about appropriate health care for specific medical conditions. Managed care organizations frequently use these guidelines to evaluate appropriateness and medical necessity of care. Also referred to as practice parameters, practice options, practice policies or practice standards.

Some organizations that have assembled practice guidelines include the Agency of Health Care Research & Policy, American College of Obstetrics and Gynecology, American College of Neurology, National Asthma Education Program, American Thoracic Society, and the American College of Cardiology.

practice parameters – *See practice guidelines.*

practice privileges – *See clinical privileges.*

pre-admission authorization – *See pre-certification.*

pre-admission certification (PAC) – *See pre-certification.*

pre-admission review (PAR) – *See pre-certification.*

pre-admission testing – Tests taken prior to a hospital admission. In some hospitals, a pre-admission testing program is available that allows a scheduled bed-patient to receive diagnostic testing workup on an outpatient basis, not to be repeated after inpatient admission.

pre-authorization – Advance notice given to and approved by the health insurance or managed care company prior to a member receiving treatment. In pre-authorization, the health insurance or managed care company agrees that the treatment is necessary. Closely related to pre-certification. *See pre-certification.*

pre-certification – A method of monitoring and controlling utilization by evaluating the need for medical service prior to it being performed. The pre-certification process evaluates the appropriateness and medical necessity of hospitalization or surgery, and determines if medical expenses should be approved or denied for the service being rendered. Also called pre-admission certification.

Pre-authorization must be obtained from the managed care company prior to the delivery of certain services for benefits to be provided and the provider to be reimbursed. Examples include surgery, abortion, and some dental procedures. Otherwise know as prior approval, prior authorization, or predetermination.

predetermination – *See pre-certification.*

P

pre-estimate of cost – *See pre-certification.*

pre-existing condition (PEC) – Illnesses or problems a patient had before obtaining an insurance policy. Specifically, a condition or diagnosis which existed (or for which treatment was received) before coverage began under a current health plan or insurance contract, and for which benefits may not be available or are limited.

Examples of pre-existing conditions may include chronic illness, injury, and possibly pregnancy. Some insurance companies may refuse to issue a policy or not pay for care for the pre-existing condition or may not pay for that condition for a set period of time. Federally-qualified HMOs cannot limit coverage for pre-existing conditions. *See federally qualified HMOs.*

pre-stenciled claim form – Reference to a service report whereby the provider's name, address, and identification numbers have been preprinted on the form.

preferred plan – A health care plan which requires the member to use one of the network's doctors for health care rather than a doctor of their own choosing if the member wishes to have a larger portion of their medical costs paid by the payer.

preferred provider – Any hospital, ambulatory surgical center, physician, podiatrist, Doctor of Dental Surgery, Doctor of Dental Medicine, or other licensed health care professional with a contract to participate in a preferred provider organization (PPO) health plan.

preferred provider organization (PPO) – A health care delivery system that is formed through negotiations between those who pay for care (employers or insurers) and those who deliver care (providers). Payers agree to encourage their members or employees to use providers who usually have agreed to supply services at a specified, negotiated rate (discounted fee-for-service). The agreement is designed to reduce costs for payers, and in return, supply additional patients to providers. Like traditional indemnity plans, some PPOs require claim forms.

Members have freedom-of-choice among in-network providers, including specialists, and are given incentives (such as lower deductibles and copays) to use providers within the network. Members may use out-of-network providers, but are responsible for a larger portion of the provider's bill, and miss out on the full benefits of the PPO plan. For example, patients who go to an in-network provider can get 90 or 100 percent coverage of their costs

P

versus patients who go outside the network.

A PPO is considered a managed care program; less managed than an HMO, but more managed than traditional indemnity. Members pay a higher premium versus HMO or POS plans for this freedom-of-choice and, usually, annual deductibles must be met before members can take advantage of some benefits. *See discounted fee-for-service, in-network and out-of-network.*

preferred risk – A health insurance classification indicating a risk that is superior to the average risk and eligible for a reduced rate.

pregnancy care – Federal maternity legislation, enacted in 1978, requires that employers with 15 or more employees who are engaged in interstate commerce provide the same benefits for pregnancy, childbirth, and related medical conditions as for any other sickness or injury. This includes all employers who are, or become, subject to Title VII of the Civil Rights Act of 1964.

premium – The monthly payment made by the health insurance policyholder (insured person, member or subscriber) to an insurance company to initiate or to keep existing insurance coverage. Also, the amount paid for any insurance policy.

prepaid group practice – *See prepaid group practice plan.*

prepaid group practice plan – A plan where a group of physicians and other health professionals contract to provide preventive, diagnostic and treatment services on a continuing basis for enrolled members. Payment is made in advance on a fixed, periodic basis (e.g., monthly) by or on behalf of each covered person. *See prepaid health plan* (PHP).

prepaid health care – A health plan where premiums are paid before health care services are rendered. *See HMO, group model HMO and staff model HMO.*

prepaid health plan (PHP) – A partially capitated, pre-paid managed care arrangement in which the managed care company is at risk for certain services. The plan provides these services to members in return for a periodic premium (usually monthly).

prepaid prescription drug program – A program that allows members of certain groups to receive reimbursement for prescription drugs.

prepayment – A method of paying for the cost of health care services prior to their use. Prepayment may be in the form of premiums, dues or contributions through regular payments (e.g., monthly).

P

prescription – A written direction or order for the preparation and administration of a drug or other remedy by a physician, dentist or other practitioner licensed by law to prescribe such a drug.

prescription benefit manager (PBM) – An organization that monitors prescription claims for HMO's and tracks the drugs and volume prescribed by the plan's participating physicians.

prescription drug deductible – An amount specified in the schedule of benefits for the prescription drug benefit that must be paid by a participant for each prescription drug or refill dispensed.

prescription drug plan – A component of a health plan where either 1) prescription drug expenses are subject to the same deductible and co-payments as other covered medical expenses, or 2) a member uses a prescription drug card (issued by the health plan) where drug expenses are covered for little or no cost.

prescription drugs – A drug that has been approved by the U.S. Food and Drug Administration (FDA) and can, under federal and state laws, be dispensed only pursuant to a prescription order from a duly licensed physician, Doctor of Dental Surgery, Doctor of Dental Medicine, Podiatrist or Doctor of Veterinary Medicine.   Only a licensed, registered pharmacist or physician may dispense the prescription.

prescription medication – *See prescription drugs.*

pre-treatment estimate – *See pre-certification.*

prevailing charge – One of the factors determining a physician's payment for service under Medicare, set at a percentile of customary charges of all physicians in a geographical area. *Also see usual, customary and reasonable.*

prevalence – The number of cases of disease, infected persons or persons with some other attribute, present at a particular time and in relation to the size of the population from which the numbers are drawn. Compare to incidence (the frequency of disease, etc.).

preventive care – A comprehensive type of care emphasizing priorities for prevention, early detection and early treatment of conditions, generally including routine physical examinations, immunization, well person care, smoking cessation and prenatal care. In short, its purpose is to prevent people from becoming sick. Also called disease prevention and health management.

previous – Refers to the category of a member who has had prior hos-

P

pital or medical surgical utilization. This is used in a system of checking claims before approval is sent to the provider of the service or supplies.

primary beneficiary – The beneficiary named first to receive proceeds from a policy on an insured.

primary care –
1. The point when the patient first seeks assistance from the medical care system.
2. Routine medical care normally provided in a doctor's office. Usually rendered by general practitioners, family practitioners, internists, obstetricians and pediatricians — often referred to as primary care physicians.
3. Professional and related services administered by a general internist, family practitioner, obstetrician-gynecologist or pediatrician in an ambulatory setting, with referral to secondary care specialists as necessary.

primary care case management (PCCM) – A freedom of choice waiver program allowed under Section 1915(b) of the Social Security Act. PCCM is a managed care option that lets states contract directly with primary care providers who agree to be responsible for all medical services to Medicaid recipients under their care, including the authorization of specialty care. Under PCCM, the state pays the primary care physician a monthly case management fee in addition to a fee-for-services (FFS). *See Section* 1915(*b*).

primary care network (PCN) – A group of primary care physicians (PCPs) who have joined together to share the risk of providing care to members of a given health plan. The structure for these networks may vary from a loose association of physicians in a geographic area with limited sharing of overhead and patient referrals to a more structured association with commonly owned satellite clinics.

primary care physician (PCP) – A physician trained to be a generalist, usually in one of the following medical specialties: family practice/general practice (adults and children), internal medicine (adults only), and pediatrics (children only). Obstetrics/gynecology (women), although usually considered a specialty, may also be considered primary care, depending on the managed care health plan.

Within managed care health plans, the primary care physician is responsible for coordinating the total health services of members, providing patients with routine medical care or referring them for specialized diagnosis and treatment. They are also the initial inter-

P

face between the member and the medical care system.

Primary care physicians often participate in teams made up of specialists and other health professionals to study and improve how care is provided, particularly for patients at highest medical risk.

primary care provider (PCP) – *See primary care physician.*

primary carrier – A health insurer obligated to pay losses prior to any liability of other secondary insurers or after Medicare's benefit payments.

primary coverage – A health plan that pays its expenses without consideration of other plans under coordination of benefits rules.

primary diagnosis – The condition, symptoms, illness, or injury that is the foremost reason for care a patient receives or needs.

primary physician capitation – The amount paid to each physician monthly for services based on the age, sex and number of the members selecting that physician.

primary prevention – Actions designed to reduce the development of a disease or negative health condition before it occurs. Examples include smoking cessation, prenatal care, hand washing and refrigeration of foods.

principal diagnosis – The medical condition that is determined to be chiefly responsible for the patient's admission to the hospital. The principal diagnosis is used to assign patients to a diagnosis-related group (DRG), and may differ from the admitting diagnosis and major diagnosis. *See admitting diagnosis and major diagnosis.*

principal procedure – The primary or main method of treating a condition.

prior authorization – *See pre-authorization.*

prior coverage – Coverage held prior to effective date under another subscriber identification number.

prior service – Information on a health plan application card of a member who has had continuous membership from a date prior to the date of the membership under which he or she is now covered. For example, a member who was covered under a Blue Cross and Blue Shield plan with his or her previous employer and will now be covered with Blue Cross and Blue Shield with his or her new employer.

private duty nursing services – Professional nursing services of a

P

Registered Nurse (RN) or a licensed practical nurse (LPN) not employed by a hospital, residential or nonresidential alcoholism treatment facility, home health care agency, skilled nursing facility, or hospice provider.

private insurance – Traditional health care coverage purchased from an insurance company. Gives free choice of physicians, hospitals and other health care facilities.

PRO – See *peer review organization.*

probationary period – See *eligibility waiting period.*

procedure code – Code number assigned to a diagnosis or service that a patient receives. Originally designed to communicate procedural data to insurance companies or other third-party payers. See *CPT codes and HCPCS codes.* Sometimes called procedural codes.

procedural codes – Same as procedure code.

product – Goods, services, benefits, or programs that are offered to health plan members for their use for a dues price. Related insurance industry terms include policy models, policy campaigns, policyholder services, agency programs, new offerings, new policy underwriting, etc.

professional component – The portion of a charge for such services as radiology, laboratory, anesthesia, or physical therapy that is allocated as the physician cost of that service.

professional corporation (PC) – An individual provider or a group of providers who have incorporated and obtained a corporate 1099 tax number, and filed articles of incorporation with the secretary of state's office in the state where the corporation is being organized.

professional review organization (PRO) – See *peer review organization* (PRO).

Professional Standards Review Organization (PSRO) – An organized group of physicians with the responsibility of reviewing and evaluating the need and quality of care and services rendered by the medical community within a defined geographic area. The term mostly applies to care given to Medicare and Medicaid recipients. Replaced by Peer Review Organization (PRO) in 1982.

profile – Aggregated data of health care services provided over a defined period of time. The data may be for specific groups of patients, diagnoses or procedures, and may be analyzed by individual hospitals or providers. See *profile analysis.*

P

profile analysis – Review and analysis of activities of physicians and patients to identify trends and assess patterns of health care services.

profile rating system – *See demographic rating.*

profiling – An evaluation of a physician's practice including patient demographics, morbidity data, mortality rates, and treatment patterns. Also known as physician profiling.

progressive rates – A method where a health plan implements new rates either monthly, quarterly or semiannually. New or renewal subscriber groups with anniversaries falling within these periods are subject to the new rates in effect.

projected costs – Claim and retention costs expected for a particular group over a future period of time.

projection factor – A factor applied to claim amounts or claim costs so they may be adjusted for assumed increases in claim costs from one period of time to another period of time.

ProPAC – *See Prospective Payment Assessment Commission.*

proposal – A formal offering by an insurer to provide insurance coverage to an employer, group, organization or individual.

propriety hospital – A for-profit hospital owned by individuals, a partnership or a corporation. Also called an investor-owned hospital.

prospective payment – A health care payment system in which the payment to a provider is preset based upon previous utilization history. *See prospective payment system* (PPS).

Prospective Payment Assessment Commission (ProPAC) – A federal commission established under the Social Security Act amendments of 1983 to advise and assist Congress and the Department of Health and Human Services (HHS) in maintaining and updating the Medicare prospective payment system.

prospective payment system (PPS) – A payment method that establishes rates, prices or budgets before services are rendered and costs are incurred. Providers are paid the established rate regardless of actual costs, and must retain or absorb at least a portion of the difference between established revenues and actual costs. Sometimes called prospective reimbursement.

prospective pricing – Setting prices in advance of providing a service as opposed to reimbursement, where the service is provided first,

P

and then the provider is paid. The Medicare prospective payment system (PPS) is the best example of prospective pricing.

prospective rating – A group rating approach that determines a rate based on a group's own past experience and projects that into the coming policy year. The carrier assumes the entire risk if the rate is either inadequate or excessive during the contract period. The purchaser pays a fixed rate for the contract period; there is no post settlement with the account.

prospective review – A method of reviewing possible hospitalization, prior to admission, to determine the necessity of hospitalization, possible outpatient alternatives and estimated reasonable length of stay.

prospective reimbursement – See *prospective payment system*.

provider – Any institution, individual, or organization qualified to provide health care to patients. Examples include hospitals, ambulatory surgery centers, home health care agencies, skilled nursing facilities, physicians, dentists, and pharmacists.

The term is also used to refer to a physician, hospital or ambulatory surgery center participating in a health plan. By participating in the plan, the provider becomes a "preferred provider" which is specially recognized to participants who enroll in that product line. Providers sign special agreements that include special pricing of their services as well as preferred treatment by the health plan.

provider excess – Specific or aggregate stop loss coverage extended to a provider instead of a payer or employer. See *stop loss*.

provider directory – A published listing of all institutions, freestanding surgery centers, and professional providers that participate in a health plan and for whose services the eligible patient member can receive the plan's level of benefits. Providers are typically listed by institution affiliation, specialty, and alphabetically.

provider health plan – See *provider sponsored organization* (PSO).

provider identification number (PIN) – A computer number assigned to a health care provider by an insurance company or managed care company to be used on all claims filed by that provider.

provider networks – Organizations of health care providers that service managed care plans. Network providers are selected with the expectation that they deliver care inexpensively and enrollees are channeled to the network providers to control health care costs.

P

provider relations or provider services – A process to service the needs and wants of providers and the education of providers and their office staff regarding health plan policies and procedures. Also known as relationship management.

provider sponsored network (PSN) – *See provider sponsored organization* (PSO).

provider sponsored organization (PSO) – A managed care plan sponsored and operated by physicians and hospitals instead of by an HMO or health insurance entity. Hence, the name provider sponsored organization. The PSO was a provision identified in the Tax Bill of 1997 that enables providers to contract directly with Medicare, allowing integrated health systems to keep 100% of the Medicare premium rather than sharing it with the HMO or health insurance company. Also referred to as provider sponsored network (PSN).

provisional privileges – Initial privileges for a provider at a medical or dental treatment facility given for a set length of time during which peers and supervisors assess the clinical performance.

PSAO – *See pharmacy services administration organization.*

PSO – *See provider sponsored organization.*

PSPM – Per subscriber per month. *See per member per month.*

PSRO – *See professional standard review organization.*

psychiatry – The study of the diagnosis and treatment of mental and emotional conditions by a Doctor of Medicine (M.D.).

psychology – The study of the diagnosis and treatment of mental and emotional conditions by a clinical psychologist.

pulmonary medicine – Branch of medicine that deals with the diseases of the respiratory system.

purchaser – The entity that not only pays the premium, but also controls it before paying it to the provider. Even though members and businesses are considered purchasers, the term "purchaser" is more readily used to describe the managed care organizations and insurance companies that reimburse the providers, because they control the premiums and are "purchasing" health care services for their members.

pure premium – The average expected cost for benefits only.

P

pure risk – Risk that can result only in loss or absence of loss, with no chance of gain.

purge – The process of removing data from the computer files.

pursue and pay – A term used to describe the adjudication of coordination of benefits (COB) provisions where the COB investigation is completed before the claim is finalized.

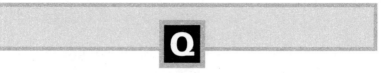

Q

QARI – *See quality assurance reform initiative.*

QMB – *See qualified Medicare beneficiary.*

QME – *See qualified medical expense.*

qualified medical expense (QME) – A medical expense as defined by IRS Code Section 213(d) that is primarily to alleviate or prevent a physical or mental defect or illness. Qualified medical expenses include:

- Medical, dental, and vision care deductibles, copayments and coinsurance
- Out-of-pocket costs not reimbursed by insurance, such as amounts above what the insurance pays or amounts in excess of "reasonable and customary" charges
- Expenses not covered by a health care policy, such as routine physicals or well-baby visits
- Any other "out-of-pocket" medical expenses that are considered eligible as a tax deduction for federal income tax purposes

qualified Medicare beneficiary (QMB) – A person whose income falls below 100% of federal poverty guidelines, for whom the state must pay the Medicare Part B premiums, deductibles and copayments.

quality – The degree to which health care services are delivered in accordance with established professional standards of structure, process and outcome.

quality assurance (QA) – A formal methodology and set of activities conducted internally by a health insurance company or managed care organization to assess the quality of services provided. Quality assurance is similar to an audit. Also called quality assurance program. *See quality improvement* (QI).

quality assurance reform initiative (QARI) – A process developed by the Health Care Financing Administration to promote a health care quality improvement system for Medicaid managed care plans. Introduced in 1993, the intention of QARI was to assist states in the development of continuous quality improvement systems, external quality assurance programs, internal quality assurance programs and focused clinical studies.

quality compass – A product developed by NCQA, based on HEDIS data, to rate health plans according to a set of performance meas-

Q

ures such as the plan's preventative care program, quality of providers, claims processing, etc.

quality improvement (QI) – Activities and programs intended to assure the quality of care in a defined medical setting or program. Such programs include peer or utilization review components to identify and remedy deficiencies in quality. The program must have a mechanism for assessing its effectiveness and may measure care against pre-established standards. In health care, QA and QI are synonymous. Formerly called quality assurance (QA), and sometimes called performance improvement (PI).

quality of life – Refers to overall satisfaction with life during and following a person's encounter with the health delivery system based on such factors as personal security, degree of independence and decision-making autonomy.

query –
1. A request for eligibility information or claims approval from another health plan.
2. Communications between a carrier and Social Security Administration determining eligibility and deductible information on Medicare recipients.

quotation – *See proposal.*

quote – *See proposal.*

radiology – Use of x-rays and radioactive materials to diagnose disease and injury.

radiation therapy – Treatment of certain tumors and disorders by means of radiation.

rate band – The allowable variation in insurance premiums as defined in state regulations. Acceptable variation may be expressed as a ratio from highest to lowest (e.g., 3:1) or as a percent from the community rate (e.g., +/-20%). The rate band is usually based on risk factors such as age, gender, occupation or residence.

rate method – The method used for billing a group, such as dues per contract type or age/sex breaks.

rate request – A request for a set of rates, based on a specified list of benefits.

rate review – A review conducted by a government or private agency of a hospital's budget and financial data to determine the reasonableness of the hospital rates and evaluate proposed rate increases.

rate stabilization reserve – Established on an account specific basis. If the account's actual experience at the end of a contact period results in a surplus of funds, these can be used toward the account's rate for the next contract year, partially offsetting any rate increase.

rating bands – Limits set on the difference between the lowest and highest premium rates to be charged to different employer groups that have different case characteristics such as age, industry and location.

rating period – A period of time, usually 12 to 18 months, that a given set of health insurance rates is guaranteed.

RBNI – *See reported but not incurred.*

RBRVS – *See resource-based relative value scale.*

re-enroll – Inactive membership re-established using same subscriber identification number; may be in same group or a new group.

real time – Processing that occurs immediately as entered as opposed to "batch processing".

reasonable charge – For any specific service covered under Medicare,

R

the lower of the customary charge by a particular physician for that service and the prevailing charge by physicians in the geographic area for the same service.

reauthorization – Approval by the health plan for extending an inpatient stay beyond the number of days initially approved.

rebill – The process of billing on a health statement for prior months' dues for dues previously billed and not paid.

recidivism – The frequency of the same patient returning to a provider with the same presenting problems. Usually refers to inpatient hospital services.

recipient – A Medicaid term defining a person who received a Medicaid service while eligible for the Medicaid program. People may be Medicaid eligible without being Medicaid recipients. *See also client.*

reciprocity – Mechanism to pay usual, customary, and reasonable (UCR) benefits for members when they receive health care outside of their home plan service area. The plan in the area where care is rendered acts as a host plan, extends benefits, and is reimbursed by the member's home plan.

reconciliation – Process of applying dues to various lines of business.

reconciliation difference code – The code in a health plan's claims & billing computer system indicating that the reconciliation process may settle a bill within an "allowable difference" and the plan can either bill or not bill for that amount during the next billing period.

reconstructive surgery – Plastic surgery that restores or improves physical function and minimizes disfigurement from accidents, disease, burns or birth defects. Reconstructive surgery is differentiated from cosmetic surgery, which is considered elective and for aesthetic purposes. *See cosmetic surgery.*

redlining – The practice of insurers denying coverage to high-risk groups.

referral – The practice of sending a patient to receive consultation and/or treatment from a specialist for which the referring physician is not prepared or qualified to provide. In an HMO, authorization is governed by the contract with the provider or health care facility.

referral authorization – A verbal or written approval of a request for a health plan member to receive medical services or supplies outside of the participating network of providers. In the case of an HMO, a referral authorization is a verbal or written approval from a gate-

R

keeper to a health plan member to see a specialist. *Also see gatekeeper, pre-authorization or pre-certification.*

referral center – A telephone bank staffed by nurses and non-clinical personnel to direct patients to hospitals and doctors, and sometimes to pre-certify or approve care. Referral centers are often used by health plans to direct patients to approved hospitals and doctors, and may also perform triage. Managed care organizations also utilize these call centers to communicate with patients and providers. Referral centers typically use 1-800 telephone numbers for easy access by health plan members. Also called triage, call center or 24 hour certification. *See nurse triage.*

referral physician – A physician who has a patient referred to him by another source for examination, surgery or a specific procedure. The referring source may be, but is not necessarily, a primary care physician who is not able or qualified to provide the needed service.

referral pool – An amount set aside to pay for non-capitated services provided by a primary care physician (PCP), referral specialist and/or emergency services.

referring physician – The physician who sends a patient to another physician or other provider of health care services for consultation and/or treatment.

referral services – Medical services, other than hospital services, arranged for by a physician and provided outside the physician's office.

refund – Dues being returned to a group or subscriber.

registered nurse (RN) – A person duly licensed or registered by the state in which they practice nursing. A license to practice nursing is required in all states, and for licensure as an RN, an applicant must have graduated from a school of nursing approved by the state board for nursing and have passed a state board examination.

RNs are responsible for carrying out the physician's instructions, providing nursing care to patients, and supervising practical nurses and other auxiliary personnel who perform routine care and treatment of patients. They also perform specialized duties in a variety of settings from hospital and clinics to schools and public health departments.

rehabilitation – A program of care that provides physical and mental restoration of disabled individuals to maximum independence and

R

productivity. Often shortened to rehab.

rehabilitation care – *See rehabilitation.*

rehabilitation center – A facility, either stand-alone or within a hospital, that helps restore a disabled individual to maximum independence and productivity.

rehabilitation hospital – *See rehabilitation center.*

rehire – A laid-off employee hired back and eligible for coverage as a result.

reinstatement – The act of restoring a canceled member to an active member status with or without continuity of benefits.

reinsurance – The practice of one insurance company buying insurance from a second company to protect itself against part or all of the losses it might incur in the process of honoring the claims of its participating providers, policyholders and covered dependents. Sometimes referred to as "stop loss" or "risk control" insurance. Reinsurance is used for protection against financial losses associated with catastrophic medical expenses.

rejection – A refusal to accept an applicant or a refusal to pay a claim. The refusal to pay a claim usually occurs because the medical service or supply is not covered under the health insurance plan.

relationship code – Identifies the sex and relationship of a member to the subscriber.

relationship management – *See provider relations.*

relative value scale (RVS) – The compiled table of relative value units (RVU), used in payment systems to determine a formula which multiplies the RVU by a dollar amount, called a converter (see conversion factor). *See relative value unit (RVU) and resource based relative value scale (RBRVS).*

relative value unit (RVU) – Basic elements of measure for the resource based relative value scale (RBRVS). Each service is assigned relative value units for physician work, practice expenses and professional liability insurance. The three added together are the relative value of the service. *See resource based relative value scale (RBRVS).*

release of medical information statement – A separate form or statement signed by the patient or responsible party which authorizes release of treatment and diagnostic information by the provider to a third party.

R

remittance advice – A form issued to a provider by a managed care company indicating any claims processed for the provider. The services reported for each patient are itemized and the applicable benefits are indicated. A composite check sometimes accompanies this form representing the total of all benefits being paid to the provider.

renewal – To maintain coverage of an individual's or group's insurance for another specified period of time.

renewal date – The date when a group may replace its present health insurance coverage with other coverage. The rates may also increase or decrease on this date. Changes may again be made on the group's renewal date, which is usually one year later.

re-opening – Re-solicitation of a group for enrollment of employees not previously enrolled or eligible.

report card – An emerging tool that can be used by policy-makers and health care purchasers, such as employers, government bodies, employer coalitions and consumers to compare and understand the actual performance of health plans. This report card provides health plan performance data in major areas of accountability such as quality and utilization, consumer satisfaction, administration efficiency, financial stability and cost control. Health Plan Employee Data and Information Set (HEDIS) is considered a report card by some companies.

reported but not incurred (RBNI) – A benefit under a health plan that is planned, has been reported to the plan, but has not taken place. An example would be a scheduled surgery.

report of eligibility (ROE) – A listing of a health plan's categories for eligible persons or eligible dependents.

reserves – Funds set aside by health plans for incurred but not reported (IBNR) health services or other financial liabilities.

residential treatment center (RTC) – A facility which can provide medical and other services for the treatment of alcoholism, substance abuse, and/or psychiatric problems to inpatients who are free from acute physical and mental complications. The centers usually operate on a 24-hour basis, seven days a week under an organized program. Most states require these facilities to be accredited by the Joint Commission on Accreditation of Healthcare Organizations (JCAHO) and be certified or licensed as such by the state.

residual subscriber – Used when an employee has a different type of

R

coverage from their dependent, and their dependent is given a subscriber identification number and billed separately as a residual member.

resource based relative value scale (RBRVS) – A Medicare fee schedule that assign units of value to each CPT code (procedure) based on the amount of time and resources expended in treating patients, with adjustments for overhead costs and geographical differences in usage.

respite care – Short-term assisted living. Respite care provides a short break for people with long-term illnesses/disabilities and their careers. Care is provided for a specified period of time and may be within a residential home or a respite care service facility. Respite care may include personal assistance for such Activities of Daily Living (ADLs) as bathing, dressing, ambulation and dispensing of medications.

restricted formulary – A list of drugs in which there are some restrictions regarding which drugs can be chosen for a health plan's enrollees to use. *See formulary.*

retention – That portion of premiums retained by the carrier to cover administrative expenses, risk charges, taxes, commissions, and contributions to contingency reserves.

retiree – A person that is no longer actively working.

retro – *See retrospective rating.*

retroactive reimbursement – *See retroactive reimbursement.*

retrospective rate derivation (RETRO) – *See retrospective rating.*

retrospective rating – A rating mechanism whereby individual groups are held accountable for their own experience (usage of health care) on a retrospective basis. Typically, gains are returned through rate credits, increased benefits or cash and deficits are recovered through a recovery factor in the rates or cash. Often called a retrospective rate derivation or retro.

retrospective reimbursement – Payment to providers by a third-party carrier for costs or charges actually incurred by subscribers in a previous time period. Sometimes called retroactive reimbursement.

retrospective review – A review that is conducted after services are provided to a patient to ensure that claims are paid appropriately. The review focuses on determining the appropriateness, necessity, quality, and reasonableness of health care services provided.

Retrospective reviews are being supplanted by concurrent reviews.

retrospective review process – *See retrospective review.*

reverse capitation – Refers to capitating specialist care while paying primary care physicians on a fee-for-service (FFS) basis.

reverse membership – Membership established in the name of a member, not previously the subscriber, with a new identification number.

review period – *See experience period.*

RFI – Request for information.

RFP – Request for proposal.

RHC – *See rural health clinic.*

rheumatology – The study of the diagnosis and treatment of arthritis and rheumatic disorders.

rider – An amending clause added to the original insurance policy that may increase or decrease policy coverage. *See amendment.*

risk –
1. The finances used for providing patient care. For example, physicians may be held at risk if hospitalization rates exceed agreed upon thresholds. The sharing of risk is often employed as a utilization control mechanism within an HMO.
2. The probability of a loss occurring within a given population.

risk adjustment – A system of adjusting capitation rates paid to providers for services to a group of enrollees whose medical care is known to be more costly than average. Higher medical costs may be due to such differing variables as medical condition, geographic location, age, gender, ethnicity or race.

risk-bearing entity – An entity (a person or company) that assumes financial responsibility for the provision of a specified set of benefits by accepting prepayment for the cost of care. Examples of risk-bearing entities include health insurers, health plans and self-funded employers.

risk contract – An agreement with a health plan to furnish services for plan enrollees for a determined, fixed payment. The health plan is liable for those contractually offered services without regard to their extent or cost.

risk factors – Conditions that influence a person's health and are capable of provoking ill health, including inherited or biological risk fac-

R

tors, environmental risk factors and behavioral risk factors.

risk load – In underwriting, a factor that is multiplied into the rate to offset some adverse parameter of the group.

risk management – Management of the coverage risks related to the financing of medical care benefits.

risk pool –
  1. The people who will make up an insured group, based on their health status, factors such as age and sex, and their predicted health. Expected losses for pools can be forecast with more certainty than unpooled individuals.
  2. State-created programs that group individuals who cannot secure coverage in the private market. Funding of such programs come from the state or an assessment on insurers.
  3. A pool of funds that are set aside as reserves to cover over-utilization or to encourage limits on utilization. The pool is determined by size, geographic location or claim dollars per individual that exceed a specified level. Under capitation, any surplus in the risk pool not used by the end of the contract year is often dispersed to participating providers. Also known as a pool.

risk rating – A rating system used by health plans to set premiums based on an individual's assessed health risk status. The idea is that an individual's health-related behavior is an indicator of high health care expenditures. That is, high-risk individuals will pay more than the average individual.

risk selection – Occurrence when a disproportionate share of high or low users of care join a health plan. It is also used to describe the skimming of healthy people by a health plan to enroll into the plan; known as cherry picking. *See adverse selection and cherry picking.*

risk sharing – A method where a health plan (usually an HMO) and contracted providers share the financial risk and rewards involved in cost effectively caring for the plan's members. Premiums are the only payment providers receive, which is intended to act as an incentive to control the costs of care. *See shared savings, capitation, withhold and risk pool.*

ROE – *See report of eligibility.*

routine – Medical procedures performed on a regular basis, such as a physical or check-up.

routine home care days – A day on which a member who has elected to receive hospice care is at home and not receiving continuous care.

R

routine newborn services – The initial inpatient examination of a newborn child performed by a physician other than the delivering physician or the physician who administered anesthetics during the delivery.

RTC – Residential treatment center (for children with behavioral problems).

rural health clinic (RHC) – A public or private hospital, clinic or physician practice designated by the federal government as in compliance with the Rural Health Clinics Act (Public Law 95-210). The practice must be located in a medically underserved area or a health professions shortage area and use a physician assistant and/or nurse practitioners to deliver services. A rural health clinic must be licensed by the state and provide preventive services.

Rural Health Clinics Act – Establishes a reimbursement mechanism to support the provision of primary care services in rural areas. Public Law 95-210 was enacted in 1977 and authorizes the expanded use of physician assistants, nurse practitioners and certified nurse practitioners; extends Medicare and Medicaid reimbursement to designated clinics; and raises Medicaid reimbursement levels to those set by Medicare. *See rural health clinic* (RHC).

safety zone – Refers to the specific circumstances that must exist for competing health care providers to share fee-related information without fear of federal antitrust violations. The circumstances can be substantial "risk sharing" among the providers, such as capitation, the use of a messenger model, or an agent that contracts for the providers independently from each other. *See messenger model.*

same-day surgery – Surgical procedures performed on patients admitted and discharged from the hospital on the day of the surgery.

sanction – Reprimand of a provider by a health plan.

sanitizing – Overwriting or erasing information so that it will not be mistakenly disclosed.

saturation – Describes when an HMO achieves its maximum penetration either in a particular subscriber group or in the marketplace itself. *See penetration.*

schedule of benefits – A section contained in the membership certificate that specifies certain limitations on membership benefits and payments, applicable to the participants under the certificate.

schedule of eligibility – A section contained in the membership certificate that lists the categories of individuals who are eligible persons or eligible dependents.

school health and related services (SHARS) – Medicaid optional benefit that provides services related to a child's individual education plan (IEP). Services include audiology, medical services, occupational therapy, physical therapy, speech therapy, psychological services, school health services, assessment and counseling.

second surgical opinion program (SSOP) – Insurance programs sometimes provide reimbursement for a consultation with a second physician regarding a proposed elective surgical procedure after the surgery has been recommended by a first physician. The program can be voluntary or mandatory. A voluntary program informs the person that a second opinion is covered by the plan if the employee wishes to have one. In a mandatory program, if a second opinion is not received before surgery, reimbursement may be reduced or denied.

secondary care – Includes routine hospitalization, routine surgery and specialized outpatient care such as consultation with specialists.

S

Compared to primary care, these services are usually short term in nature and more complex, involving advanced diagnostic and therapeutic procedures. *See specialty care.*

secondary carrier – Insurer who provides benefits after primary insurer has first provided its benefits. *See secondary insurance and coordination of benefits.*

secondary coverage – Health plan that pays costs not covered by primary coverage under coordination of benefits (COB) rules.

secondary insurance – An insurance plan identified through coordination of benefits (COB) as having secondary responsibility for payment of charges.

Section 1115 Medicaid waiver – A section of the Social Security Act which grants the Secretary of Health and Human Services broad authority to waive certain laws relating to Medicaid for the purpose of conducting pilot, experimental or demonstration projects which are "likely to promote the objectives" of the program.

Section 1115 demonstration waivers allow states to change provisions of their Medicaid programs, including eligibility requirements, the scope of services available, the freedom to choose a provider, a provider's choice to participate in a plan, the method of reimbursing providers, and the statewide application of the program.

Waivers must be approved by the Health Care Financing Administration (HCFA), an agency within the Department of Health and Human Services. *See waiver.*

Section 1902(A)(1) – Section of the Social Security Act that requires state Medicaid programs be in effect "in all political subdivisions of the state".

Section 1902(A)(10) – Section of the Social Security Act that requires state Medicaid programs provide services to people that are comparable in amount, duration and scope. *See comparability.*

Section 1902(A)(23) – Section of the Social Security Act that requires state Medicaid programs ensure that clients have the freedom to choose any qualified provider to deliver a covered service. *See freedom of choice.*

Section 1903(M) – Section of the Social Security Act that allows state Medicaid programs to develop risk contracts with HMOs or comparable entities. *See HMO and risk contract.*

S

Section 1902(R)(2) – Section of the Social Security Act that allows states to use more liberal income and resource methodologies than those used to determine supplemental security income (SSI) eligibility for determining Medicaid eligibility. *See* SSI.

Section 1915(B) Medicaid waiver – Section of the Social Security Act that allows states to require Medicaid recipients to enroll in HMOs or other managed care plans in an effort to control costs (waive their freedom of choice). The waivers allow states to implement a primary care case-management system, require Medicaid recipients to choose from a number of competing health plans, provide additional benefits in exchange for savings resulting from recipients' use of cost-effective providers, and limit the providers from which beneficiaries can receive non-emergency treatment. The waivers are granted for two years with two-year renewals. Sometimes known as a "freedom-of-choice waiver." *See freedom of choice.*

Section 1915(C) – Section of the Social Security Act that allows states to waive various Medicaid requirements to establish alternative, community-based services for individuals who qualify to receive services in an ICF- MR (intermediate care facility for mentally retarded persons), nursing facility, institution for mental disease, or inpatient hospital.

Section 1915(C)(7)(B) – Section of the Social Security Act that allows states to waive Medicaid requirements to establish alternative, community-based services for developmentally disabled individuals who are placed in nursing facilities but require specialized services.

Section 1929 – Section of the Social Security Act that allows states to provide a broad range of home and community care to functionally disabled individuals as an optional state plan benefit. In all states but Texas, the option serves only people over 65. In Texas, individuals of any age may qualify if they meet the state's functional disability test and financial eligibility criteria.

segmentation – Establishing a group health benefits program to provide coverage to a limited number of eligible employees or to provide different levels of benefits to different classification of employees. For example, union-nonunion, exempt-nonexempt, salaried-hourly.

selective contracting – Option under Section 1915(B) of the Social Security Act that allows a state to develop a competitive contracting system for services such as inpatient hospital care.

S

self-administration – The procedure where an employer maintains all records and adjudicates all claims regarding the employees covered under a group insurance plan.

self-funding or self-funded – *See self-insurance or self-insured.*

self-insurance or self-insured – The practice of an employer or organization assuming responsibility for the reimbursement of medical expenses incurred by its employees. In such arrangements, the employer can either assume all the risk, or share the risk with a managed care entity or a group of providers.

Several variations of self-insurance are possible. For example, insure some benefits and self-insure others; self-insure all benefits up to a certain aggregate claim level; or set certain individual claim limits for self-funding and insure above that level.

To self-insure, the employer sets up a fund against which claim payments are drawn, with claims processing often handled through an administrative services contract with an independent organization (see third party administrator). Since these plans are exempt from the Employee Retirement Income Security Act (ERISA) and from most regulation, they are used often by large employers. Self-insurance is also called self-funding (self-funded). Compare to fully insured.

self-pay – Identifies the individual (self) responsible to pay the medical bills.

self-referral – The ability to seek covered services without a referral from a gatekeeper.

senior plan – Refers to a benefit package offer by an HMO or other health insurer to beneficiaries eligible for Medicare parts A & B.

service area – The geographic area that an HMO or managed care organization designates for providing service to members and from which members may be accepted. An HMO's service area may be limited by its insurance license.

service benefits – Coverage for hospital and/or medical-surgical service without cost limitations to the subscriber.

service date – For health insurance the service date is the effective date of membership. If employment related, the service date is the effective date of full-time employment.

service plan – A health plan where the plan pays the provider directly and the provider bills the plan directly, except for the deductible and copayments for which the insured is responsible.

S

SFR – *See substantial financial risk.*

shadow pricing –
1. Within a given employer group, pricing of premiums by an HMO based on the cost of indemnity insurance coverage, rather than strict adherence to community rating or experience rating criteria.
2. The setting of premiums just below a competitor's rates.

shared risk pool for referral services – In capitation, the pool established for the purpose of sharing the risk of costs for referral services among all participating physicians. *See shared savings, withhold and risk pool.*

shared savings – A provision of most prepaid health care plans where at least part of the providers' income is directly linked to the financial performance of the plan. If costs are lower than projections, a percentage of these savings are referred to the providers. *See withhold and risk pool.*

shoe box effect – When an indemnity health plan has a deductible, there may be beneficiaries who save their receipts to file for reimbursement at a later time (that is, save them in a "shoe box"). Those receipts are sometimes lost or the beneficiary never sends them in, so the insurance company never has to pay. The shoe box effect is an unusual and rare phenomenon.

shock claim – *See large claim.*

short-term assisted living care – *See respite care.*

short-term disability – When a non-occupational accident or sickness keeps an insured employee from performing the duties of his or her job for a short period of time.

silent PPOs – Through negotiated contracts, providers (hospitals and physicians) give significant discounts to preferred-provider organizations (PPOs) in return for status as a preferred provider and possibly receive a certain volume of patients from that PPO. The PPO then makes its roster of preferred providers and contracted rates available to other payers and brokers for a fee. The providers' discounts are now applied to patients who are covered by an employer or payer that has not contracted with the original PPO. These patients are not subject to any incentives that encourage them to select the preferred providers. Also called voluntary PPOs, wraparound PPOs or blind PPOs.

single-payer system – A health care system funded exclusively by the

S

government, usually through taxes. The government (or the government through a third party) acts as the only insurer, sets reimbursement rates and provides payment directly to the providers. In the single-payer system, eligibility for insurance would be based on citizenship and/or legal status, not employment or income. Germany, Great Britain and Canada utilize this type of payment system. Often called "socialized medicine."

single service plan (SSP) – *See carve-out.*

single state agency – The Social Security Act requires that the state designate a single agency to administer or supervise administration of the state's Medicaid plan.

site visit – Under the Health Care Financing Administration's (HCFA) Medicare contracting program, Health Maintenance Organizations (HMO) and competitive medical plans (CMP) are monitored on an ongoing basis to review and verify statutory and regulatory requirements. As part of the monitoring process, the HMOs/CMPs also receive a site visit from HCFA within one year of contract award and at least once every two years to monitor their compliance with Medicare requirements.

skilled nursing care – Care that must be performed by, or under the supervision of, a registered nurse. Care may also be rendered by specially trained, licensed personnel.

skilled nursing facility (SNF) – A facility, either freestanding or part of a hospital, that has been certified by Medicare to admit patients requiring subacute care and rehabilitation. SNF units have transitional beds, meaning the patients do not require as much observation or staffing as acute care units. As such, SNFs are more cost effective and considered part of a managed care strategy. *See subacute care.*

small groups – Depends on each state, but usually defined as groups with 3 to 99 eligible employees.

small subscriber group aggregate – A combination of small businesses, professional associations, or other entities formed for the purpose of being considered a single, large subscriber group.

SNF – *See skilled nursing facility.*

SOBRA – Sixth Omnibus Budget Reconciliation Act of 1986. Law that states for all large group health plans, Medicare will be the secondary payer for all Medicare eligible members of the group who are not yet 65. *See Omnibus Budget Reconciliation Act (OBRA).*

S

social HMO (SHMO) – A HCFA project that began in 1982, designed to integrate acute and long-term care for enrolled Medicare beneficiaries over the age of 65.

Social Security Administration (SSA) – Federal agency responsible for determining eligibility for Supplemental Security Income (SSI) benefits in most of the states.

social worker – A professionally trained person providing social services either as a member of a health team or on a consultant basis.

sole community hospital (SCH) – A hospital that is 1) more than 50 miles from any similar hospital; 2) 25 to 50 miles from a similar hospital and isolated from that hospital at least one month a year (e.g., as by snow), or is the exclusive provider of services to at least 75 percent of its service area populations; 3) 15 to 25 miles from any similar hospital and is isolated from that hospital at least one month a year; or (4) has been designated as an SCH under previous rules.

The Medicare DRG program makes special optional payment provisions for SCHs, most of which are rural, including providing that their rates are set permanently so that 75 percent of their payment is hospital-specific and only 25 percent is based on regional DRG rates.

source document – The hard copy document (routing slip, charge slip, encounter form, superbill, etc.) from which a claim is generated.

SPD – See *summary plan description*.

special benefit networks – Special networks of providers for a particular service, such as mental health, substance abuse, or prescription drugs.

special care unit – See ICU.

specialist – A physician who is recognized to have expertise in a specific area of medicine or surgery. Specialists must seek certification in a specialty area, which often requires additional years of advanced residency training followed by several years of practice in the specialty. A specialty board examination is required as the final step for becoming a board-certified specialist. Examples of specialties include oncology, cardiology, immunology, dermatology, neurology, obstetrics and gynecology, ophthalmology, pathology, etc.

specialty capitation – Describes when a specialist is paid a fixed, cap-

S

itated rate for providing services. There are several methods to determine the capitation rate, but typically, they are based on the utilization rates for a sample patient population. *See capitation and actuarial.*

specialty care – Care that referral (specialist) physicians provide. This typically includes orthopedic surgeons, cardiologists, dermatologists and other specialists. Specialty care contrasts with tertiary care, which is more highly specialized. *See tertiary care.*

specialty case rate – The flat fee paid to a specialist to cover all services for a specific procedure or diagnosis. *See flat fee-per-case.*

specialty code (professional provider) – A numeric code which is part of a managed care company's professional provider record and identifies the particular specialty (internal medicine, cardiology, thoracic surgery) for each provider. Typically, only specialty designations as recognized by the American Medical Association are eligible.

specialty hospital – Hospitals specifically established to admit only certain types of patients or those with specified illnesses or conditions. Examples include psychiatric hospitals, rehabilitation hospitals, heart hospitals and long term acute care hospitals.

specific stop loss – *See stop loss.*

spend down –
1. The amount of expenditures for health care services, relative to income, that qualifies an individual for Medicaid in states that cover categorically eligible, medically indigent individuals. Eligibility is determined on a case-by-case basis.
2. The process of using up all income and assets on medical care in order to qualify for Medicaid.

sponsored dependent – A dependent of the subscriber who is a member of his or her household and is dependent upon the subscriber for more than half of his or her support as defined by the internal review code.

sponsored membership – A specially rated program offered to dependent children who are not married but have reached the specified dependent age limit of the parent's program.

SSA – *See Social Security Administration.*

SSI – *See supplemental security income.*

SSP – *See single service plan.*

S

staff model – An HMO that delivers health services through a physician group that is controlled by the HMO unit. The staff model consists of a group of physicians who are either salaried employees of a specially formed professional group practice that is an integral part of the HMO plan or salaried employees of the HMO.

Medical services in staff models are delivered at HMO-owned health centers and, generally, only to HMO members. Generally, all ambulatory health services are provided under one roof in the staff model.

standard benefit package – A set of specific health care benefits that would be offered by delivery systems. Benefit packages could include all or some of the following: preventive care, hospital and physician services, prescription drugs, limited mental health and chemical dependency services, and long-term care.

standard class rate (SCR) – A base revenue requirement on a per member or per employee basis, multiplied by group demographic information to calculate monthly premium rates.

standard prescriber identification number (SPIN) – Under development by the National Council of Prescription Drug Programs in conjunction with other professional organizations, this standard number could be used to identify prescribers.

standard risk – A risk that meets the same conditions of health, physical condition, and morals as the tabular risks on which the rate is based.

Stark and Stark II Laws – Named after U.S. Congressman Pete Stark (California) who introduced the bills, the first Stark laws were passed in 1989 and prohibit physicians from referring patients to clinical laboratories in which they have a financial interest. Stark II, passed in 1993, went further in detailing when physicians can legally have financial ties to health care companies. It bars physicians from referring Medicare patients for 11 types of services (designated health services or DHS) from which the doctor profits; and prohibits a number of physician compensation arrangements (e.g., a specialist cannot pay a primary care physician for referral of a patient to the specialist).

state insurance department – A department of a state government whose duty is to regulate the business of insurance and give the public information on insurance. Sometimes called the Department of Insurance (DOI).

S

state-legislated or mandated benefits – Benefits coverage that each state requires health insurance companies to offer their groups. Each state requires insurance policies sold in that state to include benefits for a variety of medical conditions or providers. Often, these mandated benefits can add to costs greatly. For example, an insurance policy may have to cover mental health or podiatry services.

stay outlier – *See outlier.*

step-down unit – A patient care unit designated for a less intense level of treatment options, nursing care and sophisticated equipment than the intensive care unit (ICU), but more than would be applied on a general care floor. The unit includes special equipment and procedures including monitoring devices, ventilator support, intravenous therapy (IV), frequent suctioning, dressing changes and ambulation.

Since step-down units are a level below intensive care units (ICUs), they are often used for patients requiring highly specialized, time-intensive nursing care; and for patients who still require medical observation following an ICU stay. The nurse-to-patient ratio in a step-down unit is higher than the general care floor, but not as high as in an ICU. Also called intermediate unit.

stop loss – The purchase of insurance coverage from a third party by a health plan or self-funded employer in the event of unexpected financial loss to the health plan or provider. In the event of a catastrophic claim, stop-loss limits the exposure for both the insurer and the purchaser. Types of stop loss insurance include:

- *Specific or individual*—reimbursement is given for claims on any covered individual which exceed a predetermined deductible, such as $25,000 or $50,000;
- *Aggregate*—reimbursement is given for claims which, in total, exceed a predetermined level, such as 125% of the amount expected in an average year.

Stop loss insurance may be specific/individual or aggregate, and usually both. *See also reinsurance.*

stop loss attachment point – The point at which the stop-loss insurer assumes liability.

subacute care – The Joint Commission on Accreditation of Healthcare Organizations (JCAHO) defines subacute care as "medical and skilled nursing services provided to patients who are not in an acute

S

phase of illness but who require a level of care higher than that provided in a long-term care setting." Care is not dependent on high-technology monitoring or complex diagnostic procedures, but requires a team of clinicians who assess specific patient conditions and act appropriately. Currently, the federal government has not adopted a standard definition for subacute care, nor adopted a specific reimbursement mechanism for subacute care.

sub-capitation – An arrangement that exists when an organization being paid under a capitated system contracts with other providers on a capitated basis, sharing a portion of the original capitated premium. Sub-capitation can be done under carve out, with the providers being paid on a PMPM basis. *See carve-out.*

sub group number – Part of an original set of numbers assigned to a group for identification purposes. The sub group number is typically defined in two characters and separated by a dash symbol from its group number.

subrogation – In employee benefit plans, the right of the employer or insurance company to recover benefits paid to participants through legal suit, if the action causing the disability and subsequent medical expenses was the fault of another individual.

subscriber – The individual (family head or employee) who meets the health plan's eligibility requirement, enrolls in the health plan and accepts the financial responsibility for any premiums, copayments, or deductibles. At times a subscriber may also be the eligible dependents covered by the health plan.

subscriber certificate – *See subscriber contract.*

subscriber contract – A written agreement that describes the individual's health care policy. Also called subscriber certificate or member certificate.

subscriber data base – Storage areas in the computer system for data pertaining to a subscriber.

subscriber maintenance – Any changes made to memberships.

substance abuse – The taking of alcohol or other drugs at dosages that place a person's social, economic, psychological and physical welfare at risk, or could endanger public health, morals, safety or welfare. Also known as chemical dependency.

substantial financial risk (SFR) – A Medicare term used to refer to physician incentive plans (PIP). An incentive arrangement that

S

places the physician or physician group at risk for amounts beyond the risk threshold, if the risk is based on the use or costs of referral services. The risk threshold is 25%. *See physician incentive plans* (PIP).

subsystem – A division or portion of a larger computerized system. For example, there may be five subsystems that comprise membership: group, subscriber, billing, reconciliation and reporting.

summary plan description (SPD) – A description of the entire benefits package available to an employee as required to be given to persons covered by self-funded plans. Under the reporting and disclosure provisions of the Employee Retirement Income Security Act of 1974 (ERISA), a summary plan description must be written in language easily understood by the average plan participant, and be sufficiently comprehensive to apprise participants and beneficiaries of their rights and obligations under the plan. The summary plan description is normally provided in the format of an employee booklet.

superbill – A commercially printed checklist type of reporting form sold to many professional providers to report their services to insurance companies. The form is normally custom-designed to include only the procedures included in the provider's particular mode of practice. However, the form is often not accepted by managed care companies from their participating or cooperating providers.

supplemental accident – Many health plans contain supplemental accident insurance that provides first dollar coverage (no deductible or co-payments) when an injury is due to an accident. Another type of accident plan pays a fixed dollar amount—$5,000 or $10,000, for example—if a serious accidental injury occurs.

supplemental benefits – Benefits contracted for by an employer group which are outside of or in addition to the basic health plan.

supplemental billings – An additional billing for a period used to bill additional members or for changes.

supplemental health services – Benefits that a Health Maintenance Organization (HMO) may offer Medicare enrollees that exceeds their basic health service requirements, as defined by the federal HMO regulations. These services may include eye exams, hearing aids, lenses and contacts, etc.

supplemental hospital plan – Plan designed to help meet a substantial portion of out-of-pocket expenses from other health care finance plans.

S

supplemental insurance – An insurance policy purchased from a private commercial company that is used to offset the Medicare coinsurance, deductible, or other out-of-pocket costs of the program incurred by the Medicare beneficiary.

supplemental security income (SSI) – A federal monthly cash assistance program for people, including children, who have low incomes, and who meet certain age or disability guidelines. In most states, SSI income limits are used to establish Medicaid eligibility. *See Social Security Administration* (SSA).

supplemental services – Optional services a health plan covers or provides.

surgeon – A physician who is specially trained to perform surgical procedures.

surgery – Any medical procedure that breaks the normal skin barrier. Surgery consists of: 1) the performance of generally accepted operative and cutting procedures utilizing specialized instruments (e.g., injections, incisions and excisions); 2) endoscopic examinations and other invasive procedures; 3) the correction of fractures and dislocations; and 4) usual related pre-operative and post-operative care, not including diagnostic services. Types of surgery include:

- *Cardiovascular*—surgical treatment of diseases and disorders of the heart and blood vessels.
- *Colon & Rectal*—diagnosis and surgical treatment of diseases or disorders of the lower digestive tract, rectum and anus.
- *General*—diagnosis and surgical treatment of disease and injury.
- *Hand*—diagnosis and surgical treatment of diseases and disorder of the hand.
- *Maxillofacial*—surgical treatment of face, teeth, and jaw disorders.
- *Neurological*—surgical treatment of diseases and disorders of the brain and nervous system.
- *Oral (teeth)*—surgical treatment of diseases, disorder, and injuries of the oral cavity.
- *Orthopedic*—diagnosis and surgical treatment of diseases, disorders, and injuries of the bones, joints, muscles and tendons.
- *Plastic*—surgical treatment for restoration of function or for cosmetic purposes.
- *Thoracic*—surgery of diseases of the chest cavity (excluding heart).
- *Vascular*—diagnosis and surgery of blood vessels.

surgi-center – *See ambulatory surgery center* (ASC).

S

surgical schedule – A list of cash allowances attached to a health insurance policy that are payable for various types of surgery, with the maximum amount based upon the severity of the operation.

surplus lines tax – A tax imposed by state law when coverage is placed with an insurer not licensed to transact business in the state where the risk is located. Unlike premium tax for licensed insurers, the surplus lines tax is not included in the premium and must be collected from the policy holder and remitted to the state.

surviving spouse – A spouse of a deceased employee that is eligible for coverage through their spouse's company group.

suspect procedure – A medical, surgical, or diagnostic procedure determined to be obsolete, of doubtful value, or appropriate only under certain circumstances. The "suspect" procedures are identified as a result of reviews and recommendations of various specialty committees of the American Medical Association. Suspect procedures are usually "tagged" for manual review by the managed care company's Utilization Management Department for appropriateness.

SVC – Abbreviation for service.

table rates – *See age/sex rates* (ASR).

TAT – *See turnaround time.*

Tax Equity and Fiscal Responsibility Act of 1982 (TEFRA) – Applies to the employer, not the health care carrier. TEFRA requires those employers affected to give each employee age 65 and over who is enrolled in Medicare, the written option of having Medicare benefits provided as primary or secondary to other health care coverage. TEFRA regulations apply to any employer of 20 or more employees who contributes to the cost of the employee health benefits program and who is covered under the Age Discrimination in Employment Act.

technical component (TC) – The part of a procedure that includes the use of equipment, facilities or supplies. In billing, procedures that have a technical component would have a modifier attached to the Current Procedural Terminology (CPT). For example, x-ray exam of ribs is CPT 71100, but if the procedure included a technical portion, the CPT would be 71100-TC.

TEFRA – *See Tax Equity and Fiscal Responsibility Act of 1982.*

TEFRA 134(A) – A provision of the Tax Equity and Fiscal Responsibility Act of 1982 which allows states to extend Medicaid coverage to certain disabled children. *See also Katie Beckett option.*

telemedicine – The use of telecommunications to facilitate medical diagnosis, patient care, and/or medical learning. Telemedicine includes wire, radio, optical or electromagnetic channels transmitting voice, data and video.

telemetry bed – A bed whose instruments are monitored from a remote location (like a nurses' station) by wires, radio waves, or other means. Telemetry beds serve patients who need continuous monitoring, such as provided in a step-down unit or intensive care unit (ICU). *See step-down unit.*

telemetry unit – An area in a hospital, such as a step-down unit (intermediate care unit) or intensive care unit (ICU) that contains telemetry beds.

temporary disability – Workers' compensation classification describing a situation in which the worker is unable to perform his/her usual duties for a limited period of time. It is expected that the worker

T

will fully recover from the disorder and be able to return to the job after a short-term disability leave.

termination – Typically, most health insurance coverage terminates automatically if dues are not paid, if the member dies, or any dependent ceases to be eligible for coverage. If coverage is terminated for any reason, benefits are not be paid for services received after the date of termination.

termination date – The date health insurance coverage ends.

termination reason – A code used as a brief explanation of a group or subscriber cancellation reason.

tertiary beneficiary – The beneficiary designation that is third in line to receive benefits if the primary and contingent do not receive the benefits of the policy covering the insured.

tertiary care – Subspecialty care usually requiring the facilities of a university affiliated hospital or teaching hospital that has extensive diagnostic and treatment capabilities. Tertiary services includes therapy and diagnosis by highly specialized providers such as neurosurgeons, thoracic surgeons and intensive care units. Often, highly sophisticated technology and facilities available only in large medical care institutions are required. *See specialty care.*

therapeutic alternatives – Drug products that provide the same pharmacological or chemical effect in equivalent doses. *Also see drug formulary.*

therapeutic substitution – When one drug in a therapeutic class is substituted for another drug that is in the same category of drugs but has a different chemical ingredient.

therapy care – The care and treatment of any disease or condition to promote the recovery of the patient. Therapy care includes radiation therapy, dialysis treatments, growth hormone therapy, physical therapy, respiratory therapy, occupational therapy, speech therapy, cardiac rehabilitation and shock therapy.

third party administrator (TPA) – An independent organization or individual contracted with for the administration of a health insurance plan. Depending on the terms of its agreement with the hiring organization (often an employer or insurance company), a TPA may collect premiums, pay claims, and handle routine underwriting and administrative functions for a self-insured company or group. The TPA typically acts on guidelines that the insurance plan establishes, and has the capability to analyze the effectiveness of the pro-

T

gram and trace the patterns of those using the benefits.

The TPA is designated as a third party since it is separate and distinct from the employer sponsoring the plan and employee participants in the plan. A TPA does not underwrite the risk.

third-party payer – Any organization, public or private, that pays or insures health or medical expenses on behalf of beneficiaries or recipients. An individual pays a premium for such coverage in all private and in some public programs. The payer organization then pays bills on the individual's behalf. These payments are called third-party payments and are distinguished by the separation among the individual receiving the service (the first party), the individual or institution providing it (the second party), and the organization paying for it (third party).

third-party payment –
1. Payment by a financial agent such as an HMO, insurance company or government, rather than direct payment by the patient for medical care services.
2. The payment for health care when the beneficiary is not making payment, in whole or in part, in his or her own behalf.

third-party reimbursement (TPR) – See *third party payment*.

Title XVIII (Medicare) – The title of the Social Security Act that contains the principal legislative authority for the Medicare program.

Title XIX (Medicaid) – The title of the Social Security Act that contains the principal legislative authority for the Medicaid program.

Title XXI (children's health insurance) – The title of the Social Security Act that contains the principal legislative authority for the Children's Health Insurance program.

token payment – A partial payment made for a service or supply item. For example, some comprehensive prepaid health plans charge $1 for each office visit. Sometimes known as "nominal" or "hesitation" payments.

total budget – See *global budget*.

total certificate membership benefit maximum – See *lifetime maximum*.

total disability – The inability to perform the material and substantial duties of the individual's occupation, or inability to perform the usual, ordinary activities of an individual of like age, due to nonoccupational injury or illness.

T

total quality management (TQM) – An operations management technique of applying sophisticated statistical techniques and using all employees to define service processes and improve the quality and cost effectiveness of health care provided to patients. Sometimes called continuous quality improvement or CQI.

TPA – *See third party administrator.*

TQM – *See total quality management.*

traditional health insurance – *See indemnity plan.*

transfer –
1. The transfer of membership from one group to another, one membership to another, etc.
2. The movement of a patient between hospitals or between units in a given hospital. Under Medicare, a full diagnosis related groups (DRG) rate is paid only for transferred patients that are defined as discharged.

transferred business analysis (TBA) – The analysis of a risk and the development of a rate for a desired level of benefits which is adequate, competitive and consistent with the experience rating method currently being used. The objective of the process is to use the prior experience information available from a group to develop a rate which is reflective of this experience level.

transitional care – Care for patients who are no longer acutely ill and require less intense care. *See transitional beds.*

transitional beds – Beds for patients that no longer need the same intensity of observation or staffing as in an acute care unit. Transitional beds are usually found in skilled nursing facilities (SNF) or observation units. *See transitional care.*

trauma – Any physical injury caused by violence or other forces. Serious trauma puts the patient at risk of death or loss of function. There are three types of serious trauma: penetrating, blunt and burns. Sometimes, other categories such as poisoning and drowning, are considered trauma. Trauma patients may also have a combination of injuries.

trauma center – A hospital equipped with sophisticated medical technology and the necessary skilled staff capable of immediately and appropriately caring for critically injured persons 24 hours a days, 7 days a week. Trauma centers are required to have a multitude of specialists and equipment immediately available at all times. Care is waiting for the trauma patient, instead of the patient having to wait for care.

T

The difference between an emergency room and a trauma center is that an emergency room does not have these specific requirements or capabilities, and may need to transfer critical patients to a trauma center for the higher level of available care.

treatment – The management and care of a patient for the purpose of combating a disease or a disorder.

treatment episode – The period of treatment between admission and discharge from a modality, e.g., inpatient, residential, partial hospitalization, and outpatient. Many health care statistics and profiles use this unit as a base for comparisons.

trend factor – An annual adjustment factor applied to total incurred claims or claim costs to represent the assumed or known change in the level of these costs from one period of time to another due to inflation and utilization increases.

trending – Methods of estimating future costs of health services by reviewing past trends in cost and utilization of these services. *See actuarial.*

triage – The classification of patients in accordance with the nature or degree of injury or illness to determine priority of treatment and ensure the efficient use of medical and nursing staff and facilities.

triple option – The offering of a Health Maintenance Organization (HMO), a preferred provider organization (PPO) and a traditional indemnity plan by one carrier.

trust fund – A money management system for employers who are partially or fully self insured. Allows a plan administrator to track the receipt of funds and payment of claims and other types of charges to the trust fund.

turnaround time (TAT) – The measure of a process cycle from the date a transaction is received to the date completed. (For claims processing, the number of calendar days from the date a claim is received to the date paid.)

24-hour coverage – Insurance coverage that removes the boundary, or part of the boundary, between occupational and non-occupational claims. The most comprehensive definition describes a complete system of medical and disability benefits available to individuals regardless of employment or financial status or whether the cause is work-related. The simplest definition describes a system that ensures that an employee's claim is covered under the correct insurance policy, that is, workers' compensation, group health, or dis-

T

ability and that there is no double recovery. There are many variants between these two extremes.

two-person membership – Membership that includes only the subscriber and one dependent.

type of contract – A classification of membership, i.e., one person, two persons or family membership.

U

UB-82 (Uniform Billing Code of 1982) – *See* Uniform Billing Code of 1982.

UB-92 (Uniform Billing Code of 1992) – *See* Uniform Billing Code of 1992.

UCR – *See usual, customary and reasonable.*

UCR reduction savings – The dollar differential between the actual charge submitted for a covered service and the "allowable" amount as determined by the top of the customary range for all usual, customary and reasonable (UCR) and UCR-based programs.

unallocated cash – When dues payments received are not allocated within a specified period of time (three days from receipt date), the group's payment status becomes unallocated.

unbundling – The practice of billing separately for the individual components of a service previously included in a single fee and described as a combined service.

uncompensated care – Service provided by physicians and hospitals for which no payment is received from the patient or from third-party payers. Some costs for these services may be covered through cost-shifting. Not all uncompensated care results from charity care. It also includes bad debts from persons who are not classified as charity cases but who are unable or unwilling to pay their bill. *See cost shifting.*

undercoding – *See downcoding.*

underinsured – People with public or private insurance policies that do not cover all necessary health care services, resulting in out-of-pocket expenses that exceed their ability to pay. *See cost shifting.*

underutilization – Occurs when providers withhold necessary services due to cost constraints.

underwriter – Usually works for a managed care or health insurance company. An underwriter assigns a value to risks and determines the conditions under which those risks may be accepted. The underwriter screens applications and compares the information with established guidelines and controls, resolving such eligibility questions as who may enroll, when they enroll, and the risk classification under which they qualify.

underwriting – The process by which an insurer determines whether and on what basis it will accept an application for insurance.

U

Underwriting involves selecting, classifying, evaluating and assuming risks according to insurability.

underwriting gain – The surplus of health insurance premium income over benefit and administrative expenses.

Unified Medical Group Association (UMGA) – *See the American Medical Group Association* (AMGA).

Uniform Billing Code of 1982 (UB-82) – A coding system primarily used by institutional providers to uniformly identify services rendered to patients by numeric code and used to submit hospital insurance claims for payment by third parties.

Uniform Billing Code of 1992 (UB-92) – A revised version of the UB-82, UB-92 is a federal directive requiring a hospital to follow specific billing procedures, itemizing all services included and billed for on each invoice. UB-92 was implemented October 1, 1993 and is similar to HCFA 1500, but reserved for the inpatient component of health services.

uninsured – People who have no public or private health insurance.

unique provider identification number (UPIN) – An alpha/numeric "number" assigned by HCFA and given to the physician for purposes of identification on forms and claims.

unit/day – Measure of medical care on a referral. For example, mental health or office visits are measured in units; a hospital stay is measured in days.

universal access – Refers to all persons having access to at least a basic package of health care services.

universal coverage – Describes a system of health care where everyone is covered, even if they can not afford it. In some cases, it may be a type of government sponsored health plan which would provide health care coverage to all citizens. The United Kingdom and Canada have national health insurance plans that are as close as it comes to universal coverage.

unmarried/married – Married refers to an exclusive contract between a physician organization (PO) or independent practice association (IPA) and a hospital system where the two contracting parties agree to work exclusively with each other. In an unmarried relationship, the hospital system and the PO or IPA work with each other, but not exclusively.

upcoding – The practice of billing for a hospital stay more expensive

U

than the one actually incurred or billing for a procedure more expensive than the one actually conducted. Coding refers to assigning a code to a procedure performed on a patient using, for example, HCFA Common Procedural Coding System (HCPCS) or Current Procedural Terminology (CPT). As such, upcoding means that the procedure was billed at a higher reimbursement level than the actual procedure performed. The Health Care Financing Administration (HCFA) claims that upcoding is one of the most common forms of Medicare fraud. Sometimes called overcoding. *See* HCFA *Common Procedural Coding System* (HCPCS), *Current Procedural Terminology* (CPT) *and downcoding.*

unreported claims – *See incurred but not reported.*

UR – Utilization review.

urgent care – Services for a condition that requires prompt attention, but does not pose an immediate or serious health threat. Ear infections and minor cuts are examples.

urgent conditions – *See urgent care.*

urgent services – Benefits covered in an evidence of coverage that are required in order to prevent serious deterioration of an insured individual's health that results from an unforeseen illness or injury.

urgi-centers – Community-based, free-standing clinics open 24-hours a day, seven days a week, with capabilities to attend to urgent care cases but not equipped to handle emergencies.

urology – The diagnosis and medical or surgical treatment of diseases and disorders of the genitourinary tract.

user ID – Number assigned for security and reporting.

usual, customary and reasonable (UCR) – The amount a managed care or health insurance company will pay for a given procedure is calculated on the UCR basis; the lesser of the provider's actual charge and the UCR charge maximum for the care. Managed care and health insurance companies usually reserve the right to determine the UCR charge maximums, and to select methodologies for making these determinations.

Specifically, the meanings for each term are:

- *Usual*—the fee which the provider of the care most frequently charges the majority of the provider's patients for the same or similar care. Usual is determined by the average fee for a given procedure the provider submits to the insurance company.

U

- *Customary*—the range of fees charged for similar care by providers of comparable skills and qualifications in the provider's general geographic area. Customary is usually the average of the 90th or 95th percentile of the charge (depending on how it is stated in the insurance policy) for a given procedure submitted to the insurance company by all the physicians in a designated geographical region.
- *Reasonable*—a charge which varies from the usual fee or customary range of fees by reason of unusual clinical circumstances involved in providing the care. The same as allowed charges or approved fee.

utilization – The frequency with which a benefit is used. Utilization is typically expressed as the number of services used over a given period of time by members of a covered group. For example, 3500 physician office visits per year per 1000 HMO members. Utilization is often used in describing hospital admissions, physician visits, prescriptions, ambulance trips, etc.

utilization management (UM) – A process for reviewing and controlling patients' use of medical care services as well as the appropriateness, necessity, and quality of that care. UM combines utilization review and case management, and involves data collection, review and/or authorization, especially for services such as specialist referrals, emergency room use, and hospitalization. Reviews can be conducted on a prospective, concurrent or retrospective basis. For hospital reviews, it can include pre-admission certification, appropriateness of admissions, services ordered and provided, length of stay and discharge practices.

Some examples of UM include:

- *Pre-Admission Certification*—determines whether a hospital should admit a patient and whether services can be provided on an outpatient basis; its goal is eliminating unnecessary non-emergency procedures.
- *Concurrent Review*—includes continued-stay review of hospital cases, discharge-planning efforts to include proper and efficient placement of the hospital patient on discharge, and case management.
- *Retrospective Review*—follow-up analysis that ensures medical care services were necessary and appropriate to detect and reduce the incidence of fraud and unnecessary services.
- *Second Surgical Opinion*—a process that requires patients to obtain an opinion from a second doctor before certain elective surgeries. Insurers rely on second surgical opinion to eliminate unnec-

U

essary surgical procedures.

UM is often used interchangeably with the term utilization review (UR), but there is a difference. UR involves only retrospective reviews while UM provides a more proactive advantage for controlling costs and utilization by adding prospective and concurrent reviews. As such, the newer term, and more accepted term, is utilization management.

utilization review (UR) – A formal review of utilization for appropriateness of health care services delivered to a member on a prospective, concurrent or retrospective basis. Utilization review supports the efficient use of health care resources. *See utilization management.*

Utilization Review Accreditation Commission (URAC) – A Washington-based, not-for-profit corporation formed in 1990 and dedicated to improving the quality of utilization review in the health care industry by providing a method of evaluation and accreditation of utilization review programs.

value health care purchasing – Purchasers and providers working together using available information to buy and sell care based on value (cost and outcome).

vertical integration – In health care, vertical integration is when one entity is involved in all contiguous stages of health care. For example, a health care system that offers patients care from the operating room though the rehabilitation process is vertically integrated because it controls continuous steps in the health care process. Essentially, health care organizations that combine their operations to increase their efficiency and lower costs are vertically integrating. As such, integrated delivery systems (IDS) are a prime example of vertical integration. *See integrated delivery systems* (IDS) *and horizontal integration.*

vision care – Coverage designed to provide benefits for preventive and corrective eye care. Insurers usually offer vision care with basic coverage such as hospital, surgical, medical, or x-ray and laboratory benefits.

vision examination – Examination of the eye by an ophthalmologist or optometrist. Vision examinations may include taking a case history, external examination, ophthalmoscopic examination, determination of refractive status, binocular balance testing, glaucoma testing and prescribing corrective lenses.

visit – A visit shall be considered as a personal contact in the place of residence of a participant for the purpose of providing a covered service by a professional health worker on the staff of the facility or by other professional health personnel under contract or arrangements with the facility.

Visiting Nurse Association (VNA) – A voluntary health agency which provides nursing services in the home, including health supervision, education and counseling, bedside care, and the carrying out of physician's orders in the home.

vital statistics – Statistics relating to births (natality), deaths (mortality), marriages, health and disease (morbidity). Vital statistics for the United States are published by the National Center for Health Statistics.

VNA – Visiting Nurse Association.

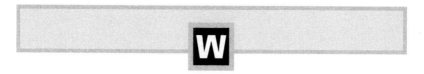

waiting period – The period between employment or enrollment in a program and the date when an individual becomes eligible for insurance coverage (see eligibility waiting period) or to become eligible for care relating to pre-existing conditions. The waiting period is usually specified in the membership certificate. Sometimes called the elimination period.

waiver – An exception to the usual requirements of Medicaid. Waivers are granted to a state by HCFA, allowing state Medicaid agencies to provide services not otherwise covered by Medicaid and to do so in ways not described by the Social Security Act. For example, states wanting to implement a Medicaid managed care program must apply and receive permission for the waiver from HCFA. HCFA granted waivers include Section 1115(A), Section 1915(B), Section 1915(C), or as home-based, community-based or Katie Beckett Waivers. *See exclusions.*

waiver of pre-existing condition – Setting aside the normal waiting period for paying claims for conditions existing prior to enrollment.

WEDI – *See workgroup for electronic data interchange.*

wellness – The process of fostering awareness, influencing attitudes and identifying alternatives so that individuals can make informed choices and change their behavior to achieve optimum physical and mental health. The overall goal is to reduce health care utilization and costs. Wellness is often introduced as programs or benefits that encourage fitness, preventive care and early detection of illness. Some examples include smoking cessation classes, exercise or weight reduction programs, and cholesterol tracking.

withhold – A percentage of the capitation payment owed to the provider that is held back by the HMO until the cost of referral or hospital service during a specific period has been determined. Physicians exceeding the amount determined as appropriate by the HMO lose the amount held back. This is known as the "at-risk" portion of a claim.

The amount of withhold returned depends on individual utilization by the gatekeeper, referral patterns through the year by the gatekeeper, groups of physicians or the overall plan pool, and financial indicators for the overall capitated plan.

The withhold system is intended to create an incentive for efficient care and serves as a financial incentive for lower utilization.

W

Typically, the withhold can cover all services or be specific to hospital care, laboratory usage or specialty referrals.

withhold pool – The total amount that an HMO holds back from the providers' payments until the cost of referrals and services can be appropriately determined. Expenditures for referrals and services that are deemed excessive are kept by the HMO. *See also withhold, risk pool, capitation or sub-capitation.*

workers compensation – A federal and state government-mandated program that requires employers to cover medical expenses and loss of wages for workers who are injured on-the-job or who have developed job-related disorders. The insurance program provides cash benefits to workers or their dependents injured, disabled, or deceased in the course and as a result of employment.

Workgroup for Electronic Data Interchange (WEDI) – A public/private partnership formed in 1991 by the Secretary of Health and Human Services to develop recommendations for government and industry relating to the advancement of electronic data in health care. WEDI's task force is made up of national health care leaders and an advisory group.

wrap around – A medical program consisting of coverage for copays and deductibles not covered under a member's regular health plan.

wrap around services – Medicaid services that are not normally covered by HMOs, but are covered by referral or direct access to fee-for-service Medicaid providers.

year – The twelve (12) months that a health plan contract runs.

YTD – Year-to-date.

zero premium – Applies to Medicare managed care plans (Medicare+Choice or M+C). Zero premium means that there is no additional health plan premium for an enrollee above the monthly Medicare Part B (medical insurance) premium required for all beneficiaries. Zero premium plans sometimes offer benefits such as prescription drug coverage, chiropractic services, vision care, dental care and hearing aids. Health plans that charge beneficiaries a monthly amount in addition to the Part B premium are not considered zero premium organizations.

Zero premium plans grew quickly after the introduction of M+C, but the Health Care Financing Administration (HCFA) now sees a decline in the number of Medicare beneficiaries with access to at least one zero premium plan.

APPENDIX

Associations

The Alliance for Healthcare Strategy
and Marketing
11 S. LaSalle #2300
Chicago, IL 60603
(312) 704-9700
www.alliancehlth.org

Alliance of Community Health Plans
(formerly The HMO Group)
100 Albany St. #130
New Brunswick, NJ 08901
(732) 220-1388
www.hmogroup.com

American Academy of Medical
Administrators — College of Managed
Care Administrators
30555 Southfield Rd. #150
Southfield, MI 48076
(248) 540-4310
www.aameda.org

American Accreditation Healthcare
Commission (URAC - Utilization
Review Accreditation Commission)
1275 K Street NW, Suite 1100
Washington, DC 20005
(202) 216-.9010
www.urac.org

American Association of Health Plans
(AAHP)
1129 20th St. NW #600
Washington, DC 20036
(202) 778-3200
(800) 631-2750
www.aahp.org

American Association of Healthcare
Administrative Management
1200 19th St. NW #300
Washington, DC 20036
(202) 857-1179
www.aaham.org

American Association of Integrated
Healthcare Delivery Systems (AAIHDS)
4435 Waterfront Dr. #101
Glen Allen, VA 23060
(804) 527-1905, (804)747-5823
www.aaihds.org

American Association of Preferred
Provider Organizations (AAPPO)
1 Bridge Plaza #350
Fort Lee, NJ 07024
(201) 947-5545
(800) 642-2515
www.amho.org

American College of Health Care
Administrators
325 S. Patrick St.
Alexandria, VA 22314
(703) 549-5822, (703)739-7900
www.achca.org

American College of Healthcare
Executives
One North Franklin #1700
Chicago, IL 60606
(312) 424-2800
www.ache.org

American College of Physician Executives
4890 W. Kennedy Blvd. #200
Tampa, FL 33609
(813) 287-2000
www.acpe.org

American Health Care Association
1201 'L' St. NW
Washington, DC 20012
(202) 842-4444
www.ahca.org

American Health Information
Management Association
919 N. Michigan Ave. #1400
Chicago, IL 60611
(312) 787-2672 x210
www.ahima.org

American Health Planning Association
7245 Arlington Blvd.
Falls Church, VA 22042
(202) 371-1515
www.ahpanet.org

American Health Quality Association
1140 Connecticut Ave. NW #1050
Washington, DC 20036
(202) 331-5790
www.ahqa.org

American Hospital Association
One North Franklin
Chicago, IL 60606
(312) 422-3000, (312) 422-3874
www.aha.org

American Managed Behavioral
Healthcare Association (AMBHA)
700 13th St. NW #950
Washington, DC 20005
(202) 434-4565
www.ambha.org

American Medical Association (AMA)
515 N. State St.
Chicago, IL 60610
(312) 464-5000, (800) 621-8335
www.ama-assn.org

American Medical Group Association
(AMGA)
1422 Duke St.
Alexandria, VA 22314
(703) 838-0033
www.amga.org

American Medical Informatics
Association
4915 St. Elms Ave. #401
Bethesda, MD 20814
(301) 657-1291
www.amia.org

Case Management Society of America
(CMSA)
8201 Cantrell Rd. #230
Little Rock, AR 72227
(501) 225-2229, (800) 216-2672
www.cmsa.org

Center for Healthcare Information
Management (CHIM)
3800 Packard Rd. #150
Ann Arbor, MI 48108
(734) 973-6116
www.chim.org

Federation of American Health Systems
1111 19th St. NW #402
Washington, DC 20036
(202) 833-3090
www.fahs.com

The Governance Institute
737 Pearl St. #201
La Jolla, CA 92037
(619) 551-0144
www.governanceinstitute.com

Healthcare Advisory Board (HCAB)
600 New Hampshire Ave. NW

Washington, DC 20037
(202) 672-5600
www.hcab.advisory.com/

Healthcare Financial Management
Association
Two Westbrook Corporate Center #700
Westchester, IL 60154
(708) 531-9600, (800) 839-HFMA
www.hfma.org

Healthcare Leadership Council
900 17th St. NW #600
Washington, DC 20006
(202) 452-8700
www.hlc.org

Health Insurance Association of America
555 13th Street N.W.
Washington, D.C. 20004
(202) 824-1600

Institute for Healthcare Improvement
135 Francis Street
Boston, MA 02215
(617) 424-4800
www.ihi.org

The IPA Association of America
333 Hegenberger Rd. #305
Oakland, CA 94621
(510) 569-6561
www.tipaaa.org

Joint Commission on Accreditation of
Healthcare Organizations (JCAHO)
One Renaissance Blvd.
Oakbrook Terrace, IL 60181
(630) 792-5000
www.jcaho.org

Medical Group Management Association
104 Inverness Terrace East
Englewood, CO 80112
(303) 799-1111, (888) 608-5601
www.mgma.com

National Association for Healthcare
Quality (NAHQ)
4700 W. Lake Ave.
Glenview, IL 60025
(847) 375-4720, (800) 966-9392
www.nahq.org

National Association of Health
Underwriters
2000 N. 14th St. #450
Arlington, VA 22201
(703) 276-0220
www.nahu.org

National Association of Healthcare
Access Management (NAHAM)
1200 19th St. NW #300
. Washington, DC 20036
(202) 857-1125
www.naham.org

National Committee for Quality
Assurance (NCQA)
2000 'L' St. NW #500
Washington, DC 20036
(202) 955-3500
www.ncqa.org

National Institutes of Health
9000 Rockville Pike
Bethesda, MD 20892
(301) 496-4000
www.nih.gov

National Managed Health Care Congress
71 Second Avenue, 3rd Floor
Waltham, MA 02451
(617) 270-6000
www.nmhcc.org

National Wellness Association
1300 College Ct.
Stevens Point, WI 54481
(715) 342-2969
www.wellnessnwi.org

Society for Health Care Strategy &
Market Development (AHA)
One North Franklin, 31st Flr.
Chicago, IL 60606
(312) 422-3737
www.stratsociety.org

Journals, Newsletters, Magazines

AHA News
American Hospital Association
One North Franklin
Chicago, IL 60606
(312) 422-3000, (312)422-3874
www.aha.org

The American Journal of Managed Care
American Medical Publishing
241 Forsgate Drive, Suite 102
Jamesburg, NJ 08831
(732) 656-1006

Business & Health Magazine
Medical Economics Publishing
5 Paragon Dr.
Montvale, NJ 07645
(201) 358-7500, (800) 222-3045

Business Insurance
Crain Communications, Inc.
740 N. Rush St.
Chicago, Ill. 60611-2590
(888) 446-1422

Employee Health & Fitness
American Health Consultants
3525 Piedmont Rd.
Building 6, Suite 400
Atlanta, GA 30305
(404) 262-7436

The Executive Report on Managed Care
Managed Care Information Center
1913 Atlantic Avenue, Suite F-4
Manasquan, NJ 08736
(732) 292-1100

Health Affairs
Project HOPE
7500 Old Georgetown Rd. #600
Bethesda, MD 20814
(301) 656-7401
www.projhope.org

Health Care Innovations
American Association of Preferred
Provider Organizations (AAPPO)
1 Bridge Plaza #350
Fort Lee, NJ 07024
(201) 947-5545, (800) 642-2515
www.aappo.org

Health Care Strategic Management
The Business Word, Inc.
5350 S. Roslyn
Suite 400
Englewood, CO 80111-2125
303-290-8500

Healthcare Business
Healthcare Business Media, Inc.
450 Sansome St. #1100
San Francisco, CA 94111
(415) 956-8242, (800) 643-7600
www.healthcarebusiness.com

Healthcare Financial Management
Healthcare Financial Management
Association
Two Westbrook Corporate Center #700
Westchester, IL 60154
(708) 531-9600, (800) 839-HFMA
www.hfma.org

Healthcare Leadership Review
COR Healthcare Resources
P.O. Box 40959
Santa Barbara, CA 93140
(805) 564-2177

The Healthcare Strategist
COR Healthcare Resources
P.O. Box 40959
Santa Barbara, CA 93140
(805) 564-2177

Healthcare Trends Report
4405 East-West Highway, Suite 406
Bethesda, MD 20814
(301) 652-8937

Health Industry Today
The Business Word, Inc.
5350 S. Roslyn
Suite 400
Englewood, CO 80111-2125
(303) 290-8500

Healthplan
American Association of Health Plans
(AAHP)
1129 20th St. NW #600
Washington, DC 20036
(202) 778-3200, (800) 631-2750
www.aahp.org

Health System Leader
Capitol Publications Inc.
11101 King Street, Suite 444
Alexandria, VA 22314
(800) 655-5597

Hospitals & Health Networks
Health InfoSource
425 Market St., 16th Flr.
San Francisco, CA 94105
(415) 356-4300
www.healthforum.com

Managed Care Explained Plus
CCH Health Law Online Library
4025 W. Peterson Ave.
Chicago, IL 60646
(800) 435-8878

Managed Care Interface
MediCom International, Inc.
66 Palmer Ave. #49
Bronxville, NY 10708
(914) 337-7878
www.medicomint.com

Managed Care Magazine
Stezzi Communications, Inc.
301 Oxford Valley Rd. #1105A
Yardley, PA 19067
(215) 321-6663
www.managedcaremag.com

Managed Care NewsPerspectives
Medical Data International
5 Hutton Centre Dr. #1100
Santa Ana, CA 92707
(714) 800-1131
www.medicaldata.com

Managed Care Outlook
Aspen Publishers
1185 Avenue of the Americas, 37th Floor
New York, NY 10036
(212) 597-0200
www.aspenpublishers.com/cmsa.htm

Managed Care Research Reports
Managed Care Research Reports
4405 East-West Hwy. #406
Bethesda, MD 20814
(800) 945-8816

Managed Care Update for Business
Advisors for Health Care
PO Box 768522
Roswell, GA 30076
(770) 993-3137
www.managedhealth.com

Managed Care Week
Atlantic Information Services, Inc.
1100 17th St. NW #300
Washington, DC 20036
(202) 775-9008, (800) 521-4323
www.aispub.com

Managed Healthcare
Advanstar Communications
131 W. 1st St.
Duluth, MN 55802
(218) 723-9200, (800) 265-5665
www.managedhcare.com/mhc

Managed Healthcare News
Quadrant HealthCom, Inc.
26 Main St.
Chatham, NJ 07928
(973) 701-8900
www.managedhealthcarenews.com

Medical Group Management Journal
Medical Group Management
Association
104 Inverness Terrace East
Englewood, CO 80112
(303) 799-1111, (888) 608-5601
www.mgma.com

Modern Healthcare
  Crain Communications
  740 N. Rush
  Chicago, IL 60611
  (312) 649-5342, (800) 678-9595
  www.modernhealthcare.com

Modern Physician
  Crain Communications
  740 N. Rush
  Chicago, IL 60611
  (312) 649-5342, (800) 678-9595

On Managed Care: Industry Information for Health Care Decision Makers
  Aspen Publishers
  200 Orchard Ridge Dr. #200
  Gaithersburg, MD 20878
  (301) 417-7644, (800) 638-8437
  www.aspenpublishers.com/cmsa.htm

Physician's Managed Care Reports
  American Health Consultants
  3525 Piedmont Rd
  Building 6, Suite 400
  Atlanta, GA 30305
  (404) 262-7436

The Quality Letter for Healthcare Leaders
  Capitol Publications Inc.
  11101 King Street, Suite 444
  Alexandria, VA 22314
  (800) 655-5597

State Health Watch
  American Health Consultants
  3525 Piedmont Rd
  Building 6, Suite 400
  Atlanta, GA 30305
  (404) 262-7436

Strategies for Healthcare Excellence
  COR Healthcare Resources
  P.O. Box 40959
  Santa Barbara, CA 93140
  (805) 564-2177

TIPS on Managed Care
  The IPA Association of America
  333 Hegenberger Rd. #305
  Oakland, CA 94621
  (510) 569-6561
  www.tipaaa.org

TrendWatch
  Alliance for Healthcare Strategy and Marketing
  11 S. LaSalle Street, Suite 2300
  Chicago, IL 60603
  (312) 704-9700

Internet Sites

ABC News.com: Health and Living	www.abcnews.com/sections/living/index.html
adam.com	http://adam.com
All Health	www.allhealth.com
America's Doctor	www.americasdoctor.com
America's Health Network	www.ahd.com
American Medical Association	www.ama-assn.org
American Prospect	http://epn.org/prospect/health.html
BeWELL.com	http://beWELL.com
CNN: Health	www.cnn.com/HEALTH
drkoop.com	http://drkoop.com
Encyclopaedia Britannica - Health	www.eblast.com/health/index.html
Family Doctor	http://familydoctor.org
48 Hours	www.48hours.net
Guide To Health	www.GuidetoHealth.com
Healthcare Report Cards	http://healthcarereportcards.com/index.cfm
Health Center	www.healthguide.com
The Health Channel	www.thehealthchannel.com
Health Forum	www.amhpi.com/default.html
Health Grades	http://healthgrades.com
Health Insight	www.ama-assn.org/consumer.htm
Health Law Hippo	http://hippo.findlaw.com/hippohome.html
Health Leaders	www.healthleaders.com
Health Web	www.healthweb.org
The Health Pages	www.thehealthpages.com/index.html
Hospitals & Health Networks	www.hhnmag.com
Hospital Select	www.hospitalselect.com
HospitalWeb	http://neuro-www.mgh.harvard.edu/hospitalweb.shtml
Intelihealth (Johns Hopkins)	www.intelihealth.com
Managed Care Magazine	http://www.managedcaremag.com
Managed Healthcare News	http://www.managedhealthcarenews.com/
Mayo Health Oasis	www.mayohealth.org
MedFacts	http://www.medfacts.com
Medical Tribune	http://www.medtrib.com/
Medscape	www.medscape.com
Modern Healthcare	www.modernhealthcare.com
National Center of Health Statistics	www.cdc.gov/nchswww/default.htm
OnHealth	www.onhealth.com
Reuters News – Health	www.reutershealth.com
Thrive	www.thriveonline.com
WebMD	www.webmd.com
Wellness Junction	www.wellnessjunction.com
YourHealth.com	http://YourHealth.com